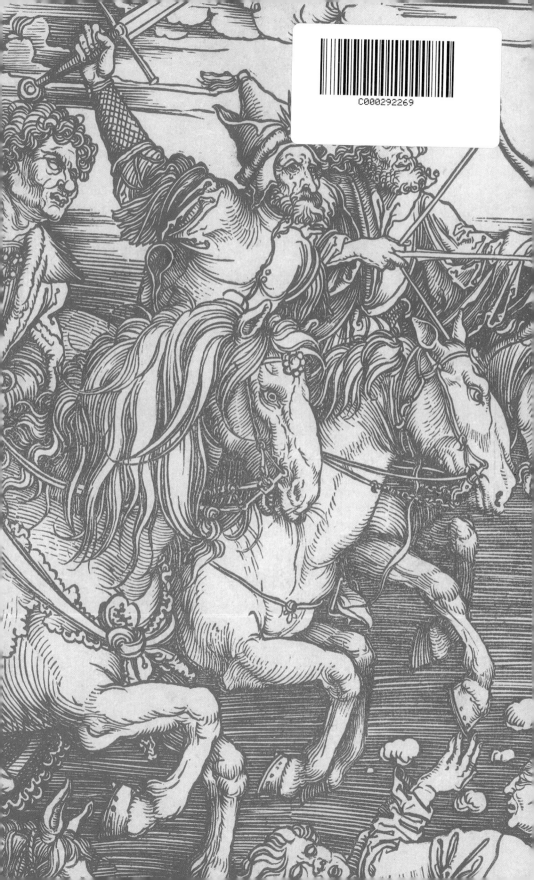

THE
FOUR HORSEMEN

THE
FOUR HORSEMEN

*War, Pestilence, Famine and Death
and the Hope of a New Age*

Emily Mayhew

riverrun

First published in Great Britain in 2021 by

riverrun

An imprint of

Quercus Editions Ltd
Carmelite House
50 Victoria Embankment
London EC4Y 0DZ

An Hachette UK company

A CIP catalogue record for this book is available
from the British Library

HB ISBN 978 1 52940 171 4
TPB ISBN 978 1 52940 172 1
EBOOK ISBN 978 1 52940 174 5

10 9 8 7 6 5 4 3 2 1

Typeset by CC Book Production Ltd
Printed and bound in Great Britain by Clays Ltd, Elcograf S.p.A.

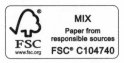

Papers used by riverrun are from well-managed forests and other responsible sources.

Contents

List of Illustrations   vii

Introduction   ix

WAR   1

PESTILENCE   81

FAMINE   155

DEATH   243

Author's Note   299

Endnotes   301

Acknowledgements   327

List of Illustrations

Page 30: Education in Mosul Under ISIL's rule: soft resistance and civil disobedience. © Mosul Eye 2015.

Page 147: Microbiologists at Kilfili Hospital researching the fosfomysin trial data, May 2020. © GARDP, Kilifi Kenya, 2019.

Page 240: Four-year-old Mahsa getting her finger marked during National Immunization Day in Herat, Afghanistan, 2018. © Tuuli Hongisto/WHO.

Page 266: Morris Tidall-Binz (right), the head of the ICRC forensic unit, together with staff from the Central Mortuary in Port-au-Prince, Haiti, carry a victim of the January 2010 earthquake to the morgue for identification and release to family members. © ICRC.

Introduction

The Four Horsemen have tracked us into modern times: War, Pestilence, Famine and Death.

Recently, our focus has been on one Horseman in particular. Pestilence bolted to the front of the group for a while, but no single Horseman is ever alone for very long. The other three are always catching up, so they can press forward together. If we need a reminder of how they ride, one of our greatest artists envisioned them for us long ago, and his image holds true and strong today. Four Horsemen, compressed into a single image, as a single group, galloping into our field of vision. In Dürer's extraordinary engraving, we see them all as they thunder past, full of detail we can relate to. Rough hands gripping bridles and weapons. Heavy nails hammered through strong hooves into iron horseshoes. Under storm clouds and across hard ground, the riders always come. We have other, newer threats to our humanity – the damage we do to our own planet foremost among them – but the Horsemen represent the most ancient of all dangers. This is a work about how we take them on in our own time – one by one, and as a company – and what it will take to stop them.

If the Horsemen have a leader, it's War, on the blood-coloured horse, setting the pace. War leads the company to the battlefield and into the devastation beyond. Into fractured cities, where sides are taken and retaken, and millions of people are trapped, besieged, dispossessed. Multiple combatants, an infinity of different forms, crashing against each other; no room for neutral ground; no firebreak to reduce the ferocity of the fighting; nowhere for those who try to negotiate, to treat the wounded, to save the children. In a world where the rider of the red horse has ended the first age of neutrality, it is up to us to envision and realize something to replace it, a second age of humanitarianism for everyone.

The Horsemen ride in our world, and in the world we cannot see. Pestilence draws its power from the microbiological universe all around us, and we usually think of it as a carrier of singular plagues. Fighting one of them can be, as we are still finding out, an all-encompassing process. But disease is only one of the forms taken by Pestilence that threatens us. We've been living in the first age of antibacterial therapeutics, and we've been drawing on this resource carelessly. While we haven't been paying attention, bacteria have been learning to fight back, enabling the evolution of a higher form of Pestilence. It's not a new species; it's a new superpower. Bacteria have developed and refined the mechanism of microbial resistance against everything we use to defend ourselves from infection.

The first age of antibiotics is ending much faster than it needs to, because War makes it so much worse. War tears open our cities and smashes medical infrastructure, clearing the way for Pestilence, making space for it to thrive. In this form, Pestilence may move more slowly than a viral pandemic, but it is inexorable. The second age of antibiotics will need to be much longer than the first, and one where both doctors and patients learn to take care alongside every medical prescription and treatment.

Famine is also finding new forms and powers in our time. Its agents flourish in the landscapes we are degrading as part of our destruction of our planet. We've reached a point where we can choose either a new age of sustainable intensity in our agriculture, or desertification. Desertification is the easier option, achieved with less clean water, more polluted soil, and irregular temperatures and weather patterns. And by other means: by War. City battlegrounds are barren. Food is scarce, unaffordable and dangerous to forage. The hungry children that live there quickly become sick children. The outcome is the wasting and stunting of families and nations. The Horsemen are once again riding together, bearing the unbearable, as they have always done. War, always slightly ahead, erodes the capability we have to deal with the agents of Famine or Pestilence, whether by its destruction of laboratories, the exile of microbiologists and agronomists, or the burning of sentinel fields.

When all the smoke and the thunder have cleared, there is always one last Horseman for us to contend with. Death is often seen as a consequence of the actions of his fellow riders, but he is there separately for a reason. Death has a unique view of us, and he often sees us confounded by his presence, particularly when the earth shakes under our feet and kills more of us than we could ever imagine. Death makes his challenge to surviving humans, and they fail it when they falter and turn away, abandoning their dead to chaos. Death understands that no human can truly live if they cannot find the means to turn back, to face him, and come to terms with their dead.

And in our own time, I think we should look beyond the original frame of Dürer's image, out into the wider landscape, to envision a new, unfamiliar point, where the Horsemen have suddenly been forced to a halt, all four of them, jostling too close together, reins pulled tight, sweat slick on the backs of their mounts, hooves scrabbling and slipping. In their way stands a line of human beings, holding fast, no matter how hard the ground beneath their feet or how dark the storm raging around them. We recognize some parts of the line already, from the work done against COVID-19, the latest weapon used on us from the arsenal of Pestilence. This is only one part of our much greater enterprise. Work is already well underway against all the Horsemen – a first and enduring response that builds on our ingenuity and commitment. This is a line held by human beings who are determined, almost infinitely varied, and interlinked, and we might miss them if we are only ever looking at one Horseman at a time. I can't show you the whole line, but I can show you some of the people who stand in it, and, hopefully, from there, we can understand their interconnectedness. To engage the Horsemen, we need to learn something simple from them, from the outset: we do our best work together.

Because it's the work I know best, I've started with a single historian, perhaps the bravest there has ever been, who stayed behind in ISIS-occupied Mosul and placed his life in daily peril to bear witness to horror. He is a historian-activist now, as all good historians should be.[1] The oldest city on Earth also sends beekeepers to the line, and architects and builders and teachers, who are putting up scaffolding, piecing together fragments of thousand-year-old carved minarets, and who seek to build a future from the foundations of the past, no matter how hard they are shaken. Of those in the line wearing lab coats to work, there are stewards of antibiotic resistance, charming and yet firm, nineteen of whom are the volunteers who walked around Damascus in 2017 encouraging pharmacists to spread the word about careful antibiotic use. There are 3,000 newly born humans and their families, who have held faith with scientists and participated in the world's largest research study of neonatal sepsis, and who will save more lives than any of them can imagine. There are professors of mycology who have loved studying moulds and mushrooms since they were eight years old, and who know that fungi are fascinating and dangerous in equal measure because of the damage they can do to our food supply, as well as to some of the most beautiful and defenceless animals around us, and to humans, when we are at our most vulnerable. Next to them stand agronomists, who have to come to the line via a long track down from the high Andes, where they have been taking pressings of wild potato species, dropping off samples at an herbarium-cryopreservation lab that saves potato DNA and is using it to create new crop varieties to feed people across our planet, and maybe even beyond. There are vaccinators, and those who seek to make their work easier with technological or statistical infrastructure. There are immunologists and geneticists who work with weight and height scales, who spend much of their time measuring the too-thin arms of wasted and stunted children, and those who work to restore what's been lost to these children before it's too late. There are peace negotiators from Finland. There are demography specialists, who've come from catastrophes where they've been counting the living and the dead, who've been there long after donors of aid have left, sitting on fold-up chairs with clip-boards on their knees, creating a space amid wreckage for survivors to answer their short, structured questionnaires, and doing it in such a way that those survivors will want to come to sit with them next year, and the year after that, and update them on their progress from survival to their life beyond. Anyone who has ever done a decent outcome study or written a really clear, focused report and made sure it is properly published is there, in the line. There are teams who deal with death in the worst of circumstances, led by forensic experts – some in hazmat suits, doing what we would expect them to do because we've seen the television series, and some in offices and meeting rooms – trying slowly and carefully to change how we think about justice and certainty, because they know that to stand for the dead is every bit as important as standing for the living, no matter where or how it is done.

Perhaps one of the Horsemen breaks away to canter along the line, to see where it ends or to try to find a way through. But there isn't a way through, because the line stretches all the way around the world, and it stands unbreakable in its common purpose. Human beings have come together in a global alliance to defend us all against our oldest, strongest enemies. They have chosen their work because they know it is urgent and necessary, but also because they find it fascinating and are enthralled by the potential it has to change lives. And their confidence in this shared purpose is our hope for a new age of humanity.

WAR

'And there went out another horse *that was* red: and *power* was given to him that sat thereon to take peace from the earth, and that they should kill one another: and there was given unto him a great sword.'

Revelation 6:4

War is used to being in front, because he has always set the pace on the battlefields and beyond. His first sight of a new line being built against him came in 1859, on the evening of 24th June, when the last engagement of the Second War for Italian Independence was fought at Solferino in Lombardy, between the army of the Austro-Hungarian Empire and the Franco-Piedmont alliance. Solferino was a proper nineteenth-century battle – light artillery, lines of infantry and cavalry – led by heads of state (a French emperor and an Italian king). It had complicated outcomes involving annexations of places hard to find on a map, and eventually resulted in Italian unification. In Europe, there was always fighting somehow, somewhere during the long nineteenth century, the Horsemen usually reaping their rewards. Solferino wasn't much different, except that in attendance was a single individual, standing a little way off for safety, waiting for the worst to be over. He was wearing a lightweight, pale-coloured suit (that legend says was white). His name was Henri Dunant, he was Swiss, and that day he was there for business, to secure a meeting with the French Emperor to sort out a land-rights contract in what would be the new Italy.[2]

Dunant had never been to a battle before, but even if he had, Solferino would have been beyond his expectations (it was technically a French victory, and is still commemorated in the name of a Metro station in Paris).[3] Both armies had marched a long way to get there, and the soldiers were hungry, thirsty and hot, in heavy, dark-coloured uniforms. They had planned to engage somewhere more amenable to combat, but Solferino was where they found themselves, so fighting commenced. By the end of the day, having endured hot sun, heavy rain, poor visibility and a lot of tramping around on a dusty, then muddy, artillery-smashed plain, almost 50,000 soldiers lay dead or injured. There were no supplies, very few doctors, and even fewer with medical instruments. And they had no means of moving the injured, so the soldiers lay where they fell. In the final hours of the battle, Dunant could only stand so much of it before he stopped queuing up to see the Emperor and stepped out on to the battlefield himself, walking among the dead and wounded, stunned by the scale of the horror, bringing what little help he could and promising to return. The wounded, he would later remember, cried out all night. There was not a moment of silence in the darkness, human voices were everywhere, close and in the distance, hoarse and choking, screaming for water, for God's mercy, for relief.

At sunrise on 25 June, as he had promised, Dunant came back. During a single night, the man in the pale suit had conceived of a plan to support those who lived and who had died on the battlefield, and he had recruited teams of volunteers from local towns to carry out the work. Led by Dunant, they fetched food and water and whatever supplies they could get. They made stretchers – because, if one constant of all wars is the wounded, the other is that there are never enough stretchers to carry them away. They cobbled together hospitals in nearby buildings and cleared spaces and found tabletops where surgeons could work. They fetched in the casualties, carefully removed the tatters of uniforms, regardless of colour and stripe, and washed their wounds to prepare them for medical treatment. They brought paper and pencils and sat on the ground beside the casualties who were awake, leaning in to catch their names and writing letters for them to their families. They made sure the letters were reliably posted. They started a process to discover who was missing and if they could be found, who had been captured and where they were being held, and who could be identified with certainty as having died. Because the dying went on without stopping for days after the battle, they dug long burial trenches and carried bodies into them, covering them with a layer of earth deep enough to deter scavengers. They wrote lists of survivors and lists of the dead, to be delivered to officers from each combatant army, so eventually next of kin would know what had happened.

On the third day of working on the battlefield without stopping, Dunant withdrew, exhausted. He would never get his meeting with the Emperor, and his business failed, but he accepted that his life had now become something else. If the Horsemen had expected the usual rich pickings on the battlefield at Solferino, they must have been disappointed. Civilians had come to battlefields before to help, but never like this, never organized to become something collectively responsible, working together. Dunant's volunteers had become stewards of the outcome of the battle – not of its treaties and negotiations, but of the humans they found there, alive or dead. Stewardship is something particular. It requires the careful and responsible management of something entrusted to one's care. It was as if the world (or at least Europe, which considered itself to be the world) had been waiting for people who could be entrusted with this work, so, when Dunant wrote his book, *A Memory of Solferino*, where he described what he had seen and what had been done, it was an instant bestseller.

In the book, Dunant asked that, the next time the princes of the military art sat down to plan future wars, or negotiate borders or treaties that might not hold, they should agree something else as well, entirely new: a convention, inviolate in character, which would create the basis and principle for the societies of volunteers who seek to bring relief to the suffering of wounded combatants. These societies should be permanent – because Solferino had taught him that battles happen by surprise, in places where no one expects them – so they would be ready to move at a moment's notice. And he asked, even though he already knew the answer, 'Is there a military commissary, or a military doctor, who would not be grateful for the assistance of a detachment of intelligent people, wisely and properly commanded and tactful in their work?'[4]

The world moved surprisingly fast to implement Dunant's recommendations. Within a year of his book, in 1862, an International

Committee for Relief to the Wounded had been set up in his home city of Geneva. In 1863, ten principles were agreed on and turned into a convention, with articles dealing with care and respect for wounded soldiers regardless of their nationality, enshrining and formalizing the principle of neutrality for medical facilities and personnel. It suggested the use of a red cross on a white background, so those giving care to the wounded could be easily recognized and their neutrality respected. In August 1864, a conference was held in Geneva, and most of the government representatives who attended signed up to the convention. The International Committee of the Red Cross (ICRC) came into existence, with its Geneva Convention as its foundation and guiding principle. The Convention's opening article enshrined its concept of neutrality. It reads, 'Ambulances and military hospitals shall be recognized as neutral, and as such, protected and respected by the belligerents as long as they accommodate the sick.' All this was achieved in four years, and just in time for the outbreak of the battle for Schleswig-Holstein, part of the ongoing process of German unification. Both sets of combatants declared that they would respect the terms of the Convention (although it would take a while longer for the Red Cross symbol to catch on).

In the centuries since Solferino, the International Committee of the Red Cross has grown into one of the largest of our world's international non-governmental organizations. Although born of war, by the end of the nineteenth century it was also sending its detachments to aid those caught up in natural disasters (and, today, we associate it equally with both kinds of catastrophes). As it grew, it revised and expanded the Geneva Convention in 1929 and 1949.

7

Most significantly of all, it broadened the definition of victims of war to include citizens living in conflict zones. Wherever the ICRC operates, perhaps the most remarkable thing about its mission is that it remains closely based on the prototype that Dunant conceived on the night of 24 June 1859, and brought into being the next day, at Solferino, with his volunteer detachments of intelligent people, tactful in their work. ICRC teams provide medical care for those at and beyond catastrophe. They keep lists of the living and the missing and the dead. They ensure reliable communication to those waiting for news, and they never give up looking for those unaccounted for until they know, one way or the other. They visit prisoners taken in war and report on their condition. They ensure the dignity of the dead and their burial.

The Geneva Convention is at the heart of the ICRC, and neutrality is at the heart of the Geneva Convention. The Geneva Convention is the basis of international humanitarian law, so the ICRC is the steward and guardian of international humanitarian law. Many of the other humanitarian organizations in our world are guided by the same elements as the ICRC – humanity, independence, voluntary service, stewardship, universality, impartiality.[5] But not neutrality. Neutrality, as a legal, principled state – Neutrality with a capital N – is the ICRC's alone, and it makes them not just different, but unique. The organization that evolved after Solferino has assumed and operated with something that looks like significant power. Not quite a state, but almost.[6] The ICRC sits among nation states, its staff write and negotiate and sign treaties – all because they have an entity enshrined in law, secured not by great swords, but by their neutrality.

And it is this envisioning of themselves as essentially neutral that defines both the first age of humanitarianism and the age of modern warfare. We may have developed new military technology and tactics, but it is the presence of this separate party on the battlefield that has really changed things: neutral non-combatants, who are recognizable, and distinguishably separate from the combatants, and with inviolate principles to back them up and ensure they are protected and respected. The establishment of the ICRC has allowed us to think that war in the modern era is somehow slightly better than before, but neutrality has simply replaced chivalry in our delusions. War never gets any better – ask the Horsemen.

There's another principle established at Solferino that we need to remember: Dunant never asked for anyone's permission. He saw, thought and came back the next day with a fully formed idea of what was necessary, and then he got it done. Dunant's taking of the initiative to provide relief at Solferino was, like everything else he conceived, eventually formalized within the precepts of the ICRC. It claims the right of initiative – to send its services wherever it thinks they are needed, in whatever form, without having to ask permission or wait to be summoned by either side. In our time, it is rare for there to be two clearly discernible combatant sides, one against the other, with the ICRC as the non-combatant third party. In 2019, almost half the conflicts it was involved with had ten or more combatant parties, and, around the world, ICRC representatives were negotiating safe, neutral passage for its missions with 425 separate armed groups involved in warfare. It's not that there can be no neutrality, it's that, 150 years after the ICRC's creation, neutrality has become a much more complicated principle. The concept of neutrality, and its application, is in transition. We do not yet know where it is going, but we need to find out, and the ICRC is the only organization on Earth capable of doing so.

The second age of humanitarianism has already begun, and everything is much more complicated this time around. Just as we know the time and location that marked the beginning of the first age, we also have a date and a place by which to record the dawn of the second: 16 October 2016, at Mosul, in northern Iraq. In October 2016, the International Committee of the Red Cross, formally and in accordance with their Convention, was asked by the World Health Organization to provide trauma care for the civilian wounded in the fighting to liberate the city of Mosul from ISIS occupation. The ICRC declined. They had made no plans to come to the battlefield at Mosul, and would not be making any until the fighting was over. It was not the first time they had decided not to engage, but it was the first time in their history that they formally declared their non-engagement from the outset. And, at this moment, we see that, in addition to the right of initiative, there is a corresponding right of refusal, no matter how great the need, if the ICRC cannot secure for its teams a neutral space in which to work. Mosul presented no such neutral space. There were too few staff, in too much danger, in a complicated military situation, where they were unable to contact both sets of combatants equally to negotiate neutrality.[7] For all that, it is their refusal that counts. The ICRC had created the legal concept of neutrality, and a new age of war and humanitarianism where it operated. Then they ended this first age, without knowing what would come next. This was the moment that a history begun in 1859 ended, and something else now needs to take its place – a new structure, that can account for human lives and all the complications there can be in trying to save them. We see this most clearly at Mosul, where everything changed.

In the beginning, there were three sites on Earth where humans gathered to live together, where the place evolved into more than the sum of its parts and became a city. Mosul is the only one to survive into our time, and the continuity of its occupation is unbroken. In its earliest form, it was known as Nineveh, capital of the Assyrian kingdom. It was huge, reckoned to have been eighteen miles by twelve miles, and densely built behind great city walls, full of residences, some large enough to incorporate farms and parks and gardens, with the wide River Tigris flowing through its centre. The banks of the river are sloping natural terraces, and the line of the city follows them up and away into the distance. The western bank rises steeply, fifteen metres higher than the river, so the view from there has always been spectacular, and, whatever the century, it's where people have built palaces. The river is too wide to be fordable, so the people who live on each side have had to build bridges to cross it, and the bridges have determined how it has grown, as have the small meandering tributaries that flow through and under the city.[8]

Ancient Nineveh fell, in around 627 CE, with the defeat of the Persian army by the Arabs.[9] The much smaller city that replaced it was named Mosul, but it was as it had always been, spread on both sides of the river, and its builders took carts out to the ancient ruins and brought back stone segments to be incorporated into their new construction. Mosulis kept gardening and farming on the soil inside their city, which had been kept fertile and productive by millennia of agricultural stewardship, and the city grew again. By 1100, Mosul was an Islamic city at the heart of the Islamic world. Halfway between Seville and Samarkand, it was a key stopping point along the Silk Road between Europe and Persia.[10]

The Silk Road brought trade and pilgrims. Pilgrims, as the very first practitioners of the art of travel writing, toured the city, looking at its extraordinary buildings. Mosul's palaces, built along the western bank of the Tigris, had prospects of the ancient ruins across the wide stretch of water, and balconies, terraces and windows from which to view them. Everywhere in the city, surfaces were layered with painted or mosaic embellishment, drawing on the traditions of calligraphy, geometry and mathematics which lay at the heart of the arts of Islam, covering every exterior – whether stone, plaster or tile; whatever material could be worked – especially those facades that could be seen above the surrounding, humbler rooftops. To see the work from the street, recognizing and marvelling at the interconnectedness of the forms, was a religious and spiritual act in itself.[11]

Ibn Jubayr was one such writer, reaching Mosul on a pilgrimage from his home in al-Andalus in 1183. For all the rebuilding and recycling, there were still high ruins of ancient towers to be seen across the river – ancient now and ancient then – and he was impressed by the number of colleges and other public amenities. But most impressive of all was the newest mosque in the city, built only ten years before he got there, in 1172, and named al-Nuri after the ruler who paid for it. Ibn Jubayr's pilgrimage memoir records that there were benches placed so visitors could rest for a while and overlook the river, and he noted that there was no nobler or more beautiful place to sit in the entire city. Rising high above him was the focal point, of both the mosque complex and the city itself: the minaret, the tower from where the faithful would be called to prayer.[12] It was forty-five metres tall, soaring over the highest palace, which was the intention, and its architects had used seven separate bands of decorative brickwork around the tight circle of the tower. It left most of its visitors speechless, including Ibn Jubayr, who gave up trying to describe it, even when he went back to the final edit of his manuscript. He simply said it was the most splendid he had ever seen, and that its patron had also commissioned a finely built hospital at the foot of the tower.

Meanwhile, in another part of the city, one of the world's first great historians worked to record the life of the city and the Islamic Empire. Ibn al-Athir, like so many of his successors, saw history as a series of military engagements, and portrayed Mosul as a fighting, as well as a trading, power.[13] Ibn Jubayr had also been impressed with the heft of the city, writing of it as 'fortified and imposing, and prepared against the strokes of adversity'.[14] Perhaps they had missed the real strength of the place: its resilience and its will to recovery. When war came again to Mosul, in 1261, courtesy of a Mongol invasion, the city was almost destroyed. But only almost. As soon as the dust had settled, building work resumed once again – great houses rather than palaces, this time, but some things never change:

the pleasure of living with a river view; the employment of craftsmen on the cutting edge, to express both their skill and the wealth of the owner. For those who didn't live in the new generation of mansions with terraces and balconies, there were picnics on the riverbanks – held to celebrate everything from New Year to birthdays to good weather and time off, whichever side of the city they lived on – and the seagulls, more poetically called 'larus birds' in Mosul, would squawk and swoop on everyone across the wide water.

Meanwhile, Mosul was gaining a new identity as the City of the Prophets. Al Jubayr was among the first of many who came to see the tombs and monuments to religious figures who had lived and died in the city on the river. Public building works were going on almost continually in the medieval period to construct memorials for notable figures from across the monotheistic faiths. Younis (who Christians and Jews call Jonah) was said to be buried on the eastern bank of the river, and a mosque was built on the spot around 1365.[15] Shrines and funerary monuments were built to the family of the Prophet Mohammed himself, mainly through the lineage of his daughter Fatima and her descendants, who were Mosulis. Others who had been prominent in the city and who wished to be associated with the holy family were also commemorated with monuments – including imams, political leaders, and the first ever monumental tomb for a historian, Mosul's own Ibn al-Athir. Mosul became a site of pilgrimage and worship, a destination in its own right.[16] And, high above it all, as ever, stood the minaret of the al-Nuri mosque.

Although, not quite as it had been. Two centuries of hot, northern winds and strong sunshine had taken their toll on the seven bands of decorative brickwork. One side had swelled in the heat, compressing the other. Other towers might have fallen, but this is Mosul, so the minaret endured – with a distinct, not inelegant lean. When pilgrims and travellers stood at the foot of the tower and looked up, it was the lean they noticed and remembered, along with the name the locals had given it: the al-Hadba (the Hunchback). The Hunchback became part of the lives of the Mosulis, as did the mosaic of mosques and religious monuments that made up much of their city. There was no special district where these were located; they were part of the community, and closely integrated in daily life, scattered across the city like the pattern of its river's tributaries. Those who designed mosques had always been flexible, fitting the buildings into whatever space was available among usually crowded urban streets. The space would be sacred no matter what shape it was, and, although a rectangle was preferred (for mausoleums and funerary monuments), many mosques were modular, blocked into courtyards and gardens with as much space as possible for the faithful to worship.[17] Therefore, mosques and monuments were to be found among the narrow streets and crammed-in houses of ordinary Mosul residents, their architecture part of everyday street life, a reminder of faith that simply required the faithful to pass by, as resident or pilgrim, to read the text carvings on the part of the exterior that they could see – because reading is also recitation, and therefore an act of worship.[18]

Centuries passed. The Silk Road lost its purpose and Mosul declined along with it, becoming a not-very-important component of the Ottoman Empire. There were fewer great public buildings constructed, but it was a new golden age for Mosul's private houses in the Old City. Heat has always determined Mosul's architecture, ever since humans first gathered by the River Tigris, because, although the river provided fertile soil and irrigation for farming, the city is hot and dry, with long sunny days, short mild winters and not much rain (and all of that is getting more extreme in our time). Violent dust storms blow in from the surrounding desert at least twenty times a year. As new houses were built on the foundations of the old, they were designed and made to manage temperatures, above all else. So, traditional houses from the late nineteenth and early twentieth century have basements and one or two floors above ground – no high-rises. They were built up close to each other, with high walls and only tight meandering alleyways between them, to scatter the strong winds and billowing dust. The private gardens and parks had disappeared into the suburbs outside the city, and the main external space for city houses was now a small courtyard, with a fountain, surrounded by plants in pots. Around the courtyard would be multi-functional rooms, with deep, strong basements used by the entire family to stay cool in summer. Thick walls blocked out the sound of the alleys close by, and ensured privacy for female members of the family. Canvas could be drawn across to serve as a roof over the courtyard, providing shade for family gatherings, and water from the fountain was used to wash down the walls and floor, to reduce the temperatures and dust. Mosulis felt a little safer, more secure in their buildings, as they almost always needed to. In the mid-nineteenth century, a British traveller came, as the pilgrims had before him, to visit the ancient ruins. As he looked at the city around him and saw the marks of inundations and earth tremors, and his local guides told him about recent plagues and famines, he saw that Mosul was not what it had once been, and noted in his memoir that 'fewer cities have faced greater vicissitudes'.[19]

In 1918, in the aftermath of the First World War, Iraq was declared a British mandate, ending centuries of Ottoman control. Over the next century, Iraq gained independence, its own maps, and an economic boom brought by the oil industry. Mosul was now officially in north-western Iraq, the capital of Nineveh province, which shared a border with both Turkey and Syria, just a short journey across the desert. People flooded into the city from surrounding rural areas in search of jobs and money. Mosul became a hub again, with a road network and new bridges, but, as its population increased, its diversity was complicated by race, clan, sect, nationality and tribe. Social pressures increased significantly as new residents squeezed into every last square centimetre of the available housing. The great physical divide in the city itself also deepened. Those who lived on one side of the river, as they do all over the world, disparaged those on the other. The eastern bank came to be richer, better organized, with more recognizably modern buildings. The Old City, on the western bank, had become very poor, the place where newcomers stayed because they could afford to go no further, at odds with its image as the traditional, historical, cultural heart of the city. No one came to admire the view anymore.

Some things never changed. In the 1940s, the al-Nuri mosque was renovated (badly, with lots of cheap cement patchwork) by the

Iraqi government, but the Hunchback minaret was left high in its place in the Mosul sky, unrestored because it didn't need saving. The lean was the same as thirteenth-century pilgrims had observed, it hadn't got any worse, and the foundations of the tower were strong, as was its symbolic value – not just to Mosulis, but to all Iraqis in the young country. The al-Hadba stood for Mosul, for Iraq as a founding centre for all human culture, and the Iraqi national treasury had put its image on bank notes.

In the 1970s, there was a conservation survey undertaken by the local Mosul government to evaluate the state of the Old City on the western bank. The aim was to produce an inventory of what was left and what was needed to save it. Nothing was ever done with the information. The inventory gathered dust in a council filing cabinet while the Old City was by turns neglected, demolished, vandalized or built over.[20] The great nineteenth-century traditional houses were sublet into apartments, and, if their tenants were lucky enough, had air conditioning installed. If not, there were other, new kinds of public buildings which offered cool, dark places to get out of the heat, and space to dream. Mosul always had many cinemas, as soon as the medium was invented, scattered across the city, and, like everything else, no matter what the complications, the city's history can be seen in their names: the Hammurabi (named after a Babylonian king), the Granada, the Seville, the Babylon, the Hadba (after the minaret), the Andalus, the King Ghazi, the King Faizal and the al Watan (the homeland).[21]

In 1989, Saddam Hussein became Iraq's fifth president. Mosul got carried away with oil money; redevelopment, road building and huge new engineering projects cleared key sections of the Old City, destroying more of its heritage than at any point since 1918. Iraq's president and military also got carried away, invading Iran in 1980 and pursuing a fruitless, expensive war, which didn't end until 1988. Then, in 1990, Iraq invaded Kuwait and was defeated by the US-led coalition. There followed a brutal decade of UN-approved sanctions, which prevented the sale of oil, and limited imports. The banknotes with the al-Hadba on them bought less and less, and the national infrastructure began to collapse. Once again, Mosul's primary natural resource became its endurance. Factional pressures in the city increased steadily. Houses sublet into apartments became houses sublet by individual rooms. By the turn of the twenty-first century, the effect of sanctions was so dire, Iraqis called them 'the siege'. Whether siege or civil war, these are fine distinctions, and unrecognized by the Horsemen, who thrive in either. Food, medical supplies, education – all became hard to come by in any quantity or quality, never mind finding an air-conditioned place in which to dream. Then came 9/11 and its aftermath. By the time of the second Gulf War, in 2003, all the cinemas in Mosul were gone.

Along with so much else. The US army had headed for Mosul as their main point of engagement with the Iraqi army, and what was left of Mosuli local government was destroyed in the subsequent fighting. The city finally fractured, turning in on itself, sect fighting sect, clan fighting clan, district fighting district. Political and religious groups were founded and radicalized just to fight each other. ISIS had strong connections to the city, Mosul being the birthplace of one of its leaders, although it was always just one among many such groups. Gradually, what had started out as an invasion by a foreign power, and then became a civil war, slowed to become something less turbulent by 2010. Many of the more violent groups fled across the border to Syria, reassembling there with a new, extremist membership from across the entire region. But order was never really restored to Mosul, which staggered along, barely maintained by a contingent of Iraqi military forces and police; almost nothing worked. In 2011, Syria shattered into its own civil war, chaos spreading out again across the region, and the Iraqi religious radicals and the forces who had taken shelter there began to think about the short journey back through the desert towards home.

Perhaps 'fractured' is too strong a word. No one ever quite gives up on Mosul, and, as local government resumed in the 2010s, conservationists stepped forward, seeing a chance to build a future that was mindful of the city's past. One of them was architect Falah Al-Kubaisy. Al-Kubaisy sought ways for conservation to be a consideration in the legislative and administrative machinery in Mosul. He asked that the great old Mosuli houses that still stood should be protected, and he identified three likely conservation areas, in which there were thirty-four such houses. He had taken photographs and inventory of these houses, and he drew this information together with the city plans and maps and engineering reports. He presented these in meeting after meeting, building something like a consensus. Slowly, over several years, the city started to understand what had been lost, and what could be saved.[22] There were conferences and articles, and Al-Kubaisy and his colleagues successfully lobbied the World Monuments Fund to put the al-Nuri mosque and Hunchback minaret on its watch list, as a start. First save the minaret, and then the city it watched over. Al-Kubaisy drew together all his papers into a book – a catalogue of the buildings he was fighting for. He used a skilled watercolourist to make images of the city on the riverbank, and threaded his book through with calligraphy from one of Iraq's finest practitioners of this ancient art of Islam.

After their success with the World Monuments Fund, the conservationists then persuaded UNESCO to agree to a project to stabilize the old medieval brickwork of the tower (easier to stabilize than fix). A visible sign of progress appeared when scaffolding was put up to the fourth band of decorative brickwork. An announcement was scheduled for early June 2014, with a launch for the project, all the relevant senior people booked to fly in to stand at the foot of the tower, press officers setting up the right angles to show the hunch of the Hunchback. But UN organization timelines tend to be long, because they are complicated logistically, and in the meantime ISIS, fresh and bloodied from their conquests at Ramadi, Fallujah, Tikrit and Baiji, had turned their sights on Mosul. The day before they arrived, there was a particularly violent dust storm, covering everything in the city. Such had been the fear of what was coming, the Mosuli Iraqi army and police forces had fled, abandoning the city to the choking dust and a relatively small ISIS force in 250 vehicles. On 5 July 2014, it was the ISIS leader in the city who stood beneath the minaret, and rather than announcing a conservation project to preserve it, a black flag was hoisted as they announced to the world that their caliphate had come.

Although, in truth, it had not. By the time the black flag flew from the al-Hadba, ISIS was in retreat from the other territorial gains it had made in Iraq since 2011. For the International Committee of the Red Cross and the rest of the humanitarian world, defeat or victory meant the same thing. Millions of people were displaced across the region, fleeing from the horror. The temporary refugee camps they had set up in response were under severe strain. Communicating with the parties involved in the fighting was a hopeless tangle. ISIS had no formal means of communicating with non-combatants (because, to them, everyone was a combatant). In any case, not everyone in Mosul dreaded their arrival. Factions and sects used the new power base to their advantage. Alliances were made, sides taken, power shifted. Soon, the passengers of the 250 ISIS vehicles were joined by thousands of others in the city of their founder, forming long lines of traffic, accompanied by men with guns watching every building – and perhaps, in among them, Horsemen, knowing there would be rich pickings at Mosul, to be taken at their leisure. War, as ever, was clearing the way.

Beyond the men with guns, there were other watchers at Mosul. There are those in the line around the world, facing the Horsemen, who do their work by bearing witness. There are new ways to do this now, in the digital space on social media, where images and words can be instantly and globally shared. Because of its clear timelines, Mosul is the first and best place from which we can understand how these new primary sources may be used, and learn how to analyse their testimony, just as, over the centuries, historians have become used to accommodating rolls of parchment, and bad handwriting, and dense gothic fonts. In the city itself, moment by moment, to show its destruction and their fear, brave young men and women testified from where they hoped would be the safety of their deep basements or other hiding places. They sent out words mostly – not many of them, but carefully chosen – and images, when it was safe to take them, learning to rely on sluggish bandwidth, pausing only when the Wi-Fi was cut off by the Iraqi government in Baghdad who controlled the service, or when the ISIS patrol groups moved on, or when they could no longer charge their devices because the power was off across the city.[23]

I chose one in particular to provide the primary source material for this work, because he is a historian, and I find the presence of historians in the line around the world such a hopeful thing. Because he is a historian, he tends to take a longer view than is usual on social media. Before the occupation, he studied the history of the Ottoman Empire, so he has a scholar's broad understanding of the context of the past. He grew up in Mosul, and he and his family suffered as the city slowly collapsed into the vacuum that ISIS occupied with such ease. Because he was committed to watching, to seeing as much as he could, he called the blog he created to report on the ISIS occupation of his city 'The Mosul Eye'. For almost two years, he stayed, and survived, and bore witness, and this was how his city and then the world came to know him. He posted his first message, in English, at 9.30 a.m. on 17 June 2014, to tell whoever was reading his posts which checkpoints were open and which were closed. Not much later, he would watch ISIS checkpoints being set up, their guards holding laptops they had brought with them from Syria, containing databases of the names of those they hunted in Mosul.

And so the historian worked in the city of his predecessor, Ibn al-Athir. The Mosul Eye formally defined his work not just as bearing witness, but as recording history, on the afternoon of 17 June 2016, after the last points of escape in the city had closed:

> What I have witnessed today is very difficult to express in writing. There are lots of fabrications and false news that have been spread by media; however, they are contradicted by the reality on ground. My job as a historian requires [an] unbiased approach which I am going to adhere to and keep my personal opinion to myself. I will only communicate the facts I see.[24]

He watched as ISIS foreign fighters flooded the city, noted their uniforms and languages. He watched them driving in new cars, and saw when their wives and families arrived. He told of how the black flags were flown on public buildings to draw Iraqi airstrikes away from ISIS bomb factories. He noted the paradox of the city being quieter, a certain kind of peace while everyone waited to see what would happen next, and he railed against those who had left them behind, who now sat in Erbil, to the east, the capital of the Kurdish Governorate, beyond ISIS reach, in safety. He listened to everything around him, and reported on rumours that ISIS was planning attacks on the monuments of the City of the Prophets, so he sought out proof. Within a week of total occupation, the historian crossed the city to witness the destruction and complete removal of the tomb of the other great chronicler of the city, Ibn al-Athir. Then, Mosul's most famous tomb of all: 'Prophet Younis shrine completely destroyed and the Assyrian remains underneath are in danger; expectation of Prophet Seth's shrine bombing tomorrow; ISIS is in charge of the Museum now; Niqab was imposed on women today . . .'

Then, day by day, tombs, mosques and funerary monuments were not just destroyed, but erased from the face of the Earth that had grounded them for so long in the City of Prophets. Every statue torn down, its remnants taken away and blown to shards. The carefully sited monuments and mosques, closely integrated with the narrow streets and tightly packed buildings around them, were now thoroughly and painstakingly obliterated, leaving behind only a footprint visible from satellites high above the Earth.[25] We're familiar with the destruction of Christian and Jewish sites in the city, because they were reported on global news outlets, but none of them were ever attacked with quite the same detailed deliberation as these many smaller sites, most only of significance to the local population. No images were uploaded for the world to witness. Only the locals saw what happened, watching as the heart was almost surgically excised from their neighbourhoods. And, because the historian tells us the dates and times very precisely, we know that this is what they did first. That their priority was to come to Mosul and, as an act of their faith, destroy, obliterate, terrify.

Their next priority was to destroy the sects in the city whose faith didn't match their own.[26] In September 2014, the historian wrote of hearing how there was a massacre to happen soon to the Yazidi residents . . . especially that ISIS treats Yazidis by the principle 'death or Islam' without a third option. There is news too which says that ISIS had spread flyers which say that Yazidi residents don't have any choice except 'slaughter'. I must point out here that Al-Qaeda had committed terrible and awful massacres against Yazidis in the previous years which caused all the Yazidis to migrate from Mosul and they completely emptied it.

And then: 'Yazidis are forced to declare their "Islam" in order to secure safety, water and food to their children and families after they were left without any place to go, alone on the mountain.'[27]

There were breaks in his transmissions, 'due to technical and other security reasons', but he kept working into the second year of occupation, with a renewed sense of the importance of keeping a record, working with others, conscious now of the scale of the brutality and of the need for it to be recognized somehow: 'We put out this document for the United Nations, Amnesty International, Human Rights organizations, and to all whom it may concern and request to hold those criminals accountable for their crimes and consider those crimes war crimes according to the international law.'

He couldn't see everything that happened, but he saw pieces of the new, ugly mosaic that had become Mosul's daily life. He saw the motorcycles that sped around the narrow alleyways of the city, constantly stopping, searching, snatching away people who never came back. He knew civil servants, from doctors to teachers, who showed up for work and tried to cover for colleagues who had fled.

He looked at weather reports and saw the temperatures would rise, realizing that, with only intermittent power and very little water, Mosulis would struggle to keep cool, stay safe and would be forced to choose whether to use their water for drinking, washing or flushing their toilets. Eventually, the water purification system was destroyed, so there were even greater demands on income to buy it bottled, or to buy kerosene gas, which cost more every day, in order to boil pots on stoves. Drawing water from the Tigris, as humans in the river valley had always done, became dangerous, because ISIS snipers operated there constantly. Everyone felt the effects of dirty, insufficient water, and everyone saw the effect on children, in particular, who suffered skin rashes and scabbing from the waterborne parasites and their inability to keep clean.

The historian was the first to describe the ISIS economy, based on the creation of a revenue stream from taxes on Mosulis. The (digital) banking system never quite collapsed, so public-service wages were paid by the Iraqi central government and then garnished by ISIS, who took a third off the top, in addition to other taxes levied across the city. There was a 10 per cent tax on all agricultural production, and constant, random, ever-increasing fines, and the penalty for non-compliance was death, so people had started selling off their property to somehow find the money. ISIS themselves needed funding for all the new vehicles in which they drove around the city, so anything that could be traded to fund the caliphate was sold: from museum artefacts to machinery in factories and utility plants. For anyone else in Mosul, unless they found favour in the caliphate, keeping out of their way and making a living became almost impossible, without basic services. This was life under the madness of a system that banned the manufacture of pickles – a local favourite and staple in times of food insecurity, that didn't need to be kept in a fridge – because pickling juice might be used to make alcoholic drinks.

Everywhere the historian went, he met the injured, or the families of the injured and of the sick, and heard how little could be done for them. Hospitals had been hit particularly hard. The radiological units were burned, along with the medical-waste facilities. Maternity units were shut down. Health workers, who continued to try to work, were forbidden to speak to persons of the opposite sex, and the Hesba morality police, who patrolled the streets, also roamed the hospital corridors to enforce the ruling. Female medics were briefly allowed to work in the hospital during daylight to treat female patients, but only if they wore thick black robes, and they were only allowed to lift the gauze covering their eyes to insert intravenous lines. Male medics were forced to grow long beards. There were no computers, televisions or mobile phones allowed in the hospital buildings, so every time someone was needed, they had to be fetched. Most of the relatively new medical school's students had fled to complete their studies in Erbil, but a year's worth had been left behind. From then on, their teaching modules were mostly what would elsewhere be called 'austere medicine'. Increasingly, the city's hospitals became field hospitals – not just because their kit and supplies were limited, but because most of their patients were injured ISIS fighters. Few of them spoke any language Mosuli medics understood. Some medics escaped, heading for the emergency medical teams elsewhere in the region, to help with the struggling humanitarian effort or to train those who had begun to prepare to battle for the city and its soul.[28] Gradually, Mosul's civilians learned not to go to what remained of their hospitals, and relied upon mostly private primary-health clinics, informal sources (medics hiding at home) and pharmacies.[29] And, in the meantime, doctors were executed for violating the ISIS gender separation laws, or for showing reluctance to prioritize the treatment of ISIS fighters above their few, very sick other patients.

And the historian noticed a very quiet but steady form of civil disobedience. Before ISIS, 80 per cent of Mosuli children went to school. During the occupation, this went down to 2 per cent, despite fines levied on schools and families, and threats to teachers who did not comply with ISIS orders. But families did not want to send their sons to attend classes using an ISIS-approved curriculum, including weapons training and physical fitness, with regular visits from ISIS press gangs. University and school buildings were all but abandoned, as staff and students stayed away. Although the historian never liked to see anyone miss out on educational opportunities, he observed that

> ... ISIS is unable to force the students to attend their college; attendance is almost zero, and attendance is now exclusive to the academic staff appointed to the committees for rewriting the educational curricula at the main library building, and [a] very limited number of students, along with other students and graduates who visit the university for their paperwork. After 12.00 p.m., the university becomes empty of civilians and only ISIS fighters are seen scattered throughout the university.

The historian and a group of his fellow citizen-journalists felt so strongly about what was happening (or not happening) that they produced a special report for the Mosul Eye blog, *Education in Mosul Under ISIL's Rule: Soft Resistance and Civil Disobedience*, full of colour photographs of empty education buildings.[30] For its cover, they used a photograph of a female student, purposefully off to school, in a pink cardigan, breakfast pastry in one hand and exercise books in the other. In the real city, such a sight was impossible. Girls had been excluded immediately from all aspects of public life in Mosul. The morality police went to Mosul's clothing factories to ensure that only approved female clothing was being manufactured. Fleeing the city to protect daughters from forced marriages became a dangerous necessity as the first year of the occupation passed into the second, and children became adolescents, and ISIS came for them.

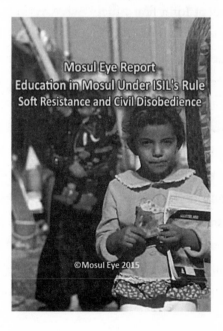

Early in the occupation, the historian heard talk that ISIS had gone to the oil refinery near the city and was planning something there. Once again, the rumours were right. ISIS ran what the UN environment agency would eventually call 'artisanal oil wells' – where they attached loading stations to pipelines to siphon off oil and sell it or refine it themselves. In June 2016, they set fire to eighteen oil wells outside the city, which burned steadily for nine months, thick black smoke darkening the skies around. Locals referred to it as the 'ISIS winter'. The smoke brought toxic fumes and dust down alleyways and into homes and courtyards. ISIS set fire to anything that would burn, and the pollution leached into the Tigris, killing livestock downstream in the agricultural areas. Sheep suffered in particular, starved or poisoned as their fleeces were covered in soot and their grazing areas were devastated. Irrigation systems were destroyed so crops failed, except for a few which were sold or stolen. Summers under ISIS were hot, and the heat was made worse because the lack of electricity meant no air conditioning or fans, and the poisoning of the river limited its use as a cooling wash-down for dwellings. Oil from damaged wells flowed down the streets of settlements just outside Mosul, and leached into the ground, leaving behind a thick crust of something – no one was quite sure what.[31] One of the world's largest sulphur mines is to be found at Mishraq, a very short distance from Mosul. It's more than a mine, it's a 'sulphur complex' – mine, sulphuric acid processing plant, stockpiles of purified sulphur and adjacent waste piles. No matter what it was, ISIS set it on fire, and the resulting thick white toxic cloud floated 400 kilometres, to Baghdad and beyond, and the stream of melting sulphur flowed into a large canal that feeds the Tigris, and eventually down to the groundwater, along with the residues of the artisanally refined oil. Mosul was already suffering the effects of desertification before ISIS arrived, its water table sinking, the dry sand encroaching further and further into what had once been good, fertile arable land. Now, the valley that once cradled human civilization was almost beyond recognition – savaged and poisoned and bleak.

The historian continued to walk around the city for hours at a time, to witness what, by then, he could only call 'ISIS absurdity'. When he came home, he rested in a chair and lit a candle, preferring to use the scarce electricity to listen to recordings of Menuhin or Perlman playing Mozart's Violin Concerto No. 3, or Mussorgsky's 'Pictures at an Exhibition'. The music reminded him that there was beauty to be found even among the ruins, and he dreamed of the day that Mosul would have an opera house, and a music and ballet school. He dreamed of sculptures spreading across the city, instead of rubble, of statues and monuments returning, a city of prophets and of art, and he reminded himself how, no matter what happened, he had fought back, with words and music and perseverance, mostly alone, with no idea who was listening. He wasn't the only witness calling out from Mosul. Others were joining him, starting up their own blogs or uploading footage to YouTube, when they could, sometimes just a few minutes' worth of film showing the larus birds flying and squawking over the Tigris, as they had always done, as they would always do, no matter who ruled the city.

Beyond the river valley, by the end of 2015, storm clouds gathered
to the south and west. Territory was being shaken loose from the
grip of the caliphate by a coalition of Iraqi and international forces.
Everyone in Mosul, occupier or citizen, knew that they were next.
The streets were almost empty, there was very little water, and
ISIS violence grew more frenzied as they waited for what was now
becoming the inevitable. Even the historian began to dare to hope:

> Get ready and dress up for your liberation, and have your razors
> ready, for ISIL and its beard will be taken off of Mosul, and we'll
> decorate its streets with the flags of civilization and peace . . . The
> churches' bells will ring again in Mosul, and we'll sing the songs
> of peace out loud . . . We'll never let the speeches of death and evil
> and the minarets of destruction rise up again in Mosul . . . We'll
> replace the black flags with colourful ones. This winter won't be
> cold. It will be warm with candles lighting up the churches and
> the streets.

In posts written during the same week, he noted increasingly heavy
airstrikes on the city, killing both ISIS and civilians – a warning that
liberation would be, as it has always been, the last and bloodiest
part of war.[32] The airstrikes were a preliminary; the liberation of
Mosul was to come by land, and its leadership would be local. Iraqi
forces would be liberating Iraqi citizens and taking back control of
an Iraqi city.[33] But not on their own. They were supported by an
integrated advise-and-assist network, primarily of US military forces,
along with eighteen other coalition partners, including the UK, who

provided force generation effort (training, preparing and equipping their Iraqi partners for combat).[34] The coalition had been working together for a while to fight back against ISIS (Operation Inherent Resolve, tagline: 'One Mission, Many Nations'). Getting everyone together, from the Kurdish Regional Government to the heads of the various Iraqi ministries and militias, had been almost impossible, but they had done it, eventually mustering a force of 94,000, made up of the Iraq army, federal police and counterterrorism units, and the Kurdish Peshmerga forces.

Lessons had been learned from the liberations of Ramadi, Tikrit and Fallujah. The liberators would face the equivalent of heavily armed light infantry, mobile, with elaborate systems of defensive works inside the city, fortified buildings, underground shelters and tunnels, a seemingly infinite number of explosive devices and the use of civilians as human shields – the dreaded 'dense urban environment' of current military-school textbooks. All those narrow alleyways leading in and out and beneath the rubble. To enable the liberators to move forward quickly, on multiple fronts, simultaneously, the plan envisaged the city as a cartwheel. Each segment was allocated to a separate part of the Iraqi forces and their coalition partners. The city would be encircled. Then, segment by segment, ISIS would be rolled up, compressed into smaller and smaller spaces, and finally defeated. As each section pushed in along their separate avenues of advance, they would use multiple firing platforms – rockets, mortars, heavy and light guns – and integrated electronic warfare equipment to try to jam enemy communications. Leaflets would be dropped to warn citizens of what they could expect. There would be teams ready to build bridges, metaphorically and literally, for when the forces crossed the river from east to west. There would be armoured bulldozers. Everyone was heading for the same operational objective at the hub of the cartwheel: the al-Nuri mosque and the al-Hadba minaret. The Hunchback tower was still standing, even though everyone in the city thought surely it would have been destroyed somehow, but every time the smoke cleared from an air or artillery strike, there it was, and it didn't even take a full motion video platform attached to a drone to make it out, just someone looking up for it every day, as had been done across centuries.[35]

If the sight of the Hunchback minaret has been the constant of Mosul throughout its history, then the constant of all warfare, no matter what the time or strategy, is wounding. At Mosul, the plan to fight in dense urban environments, compressing the enemy into smaller and smaller spaces, would mean many wounded for every step forward. We are still working out what the best military medical response to this is within well-resourced systems, but at Mosul, there was no system to start with, never mind a well-resourced one. All that time and effort spent putting together a coalition, planning a liberation in the most dangerous kind of war fighting known to humans, and it was led by a military force with almost no ability to treat their own casualties. Since 2003, nearly all Iraqi military medics had been lost, purged, driven out in political infighting or killed in actual fighting during the country's civil war.[36] By the time the Mosul assault was planned, they had still not been replaced. The main army would go to liberate Mosul with a few combat medical teams, who had not had very advanced training, and some basic medical supplies. They couldn't provide primary care for their troops, let alone casualty care. Foreign military forces had brought their own medical teams, proportional to the size of their own military's commitment. They were not planning, nor were they resourced to accept Iraqi military casualties, although there should have been no need. Each coalition partner should have been able to look after its own. But, somehow, as Iraqi military capability was rebuilt after 2003, its medical incapability was overlooked. Operation Inherent Resolve cost $14.3 billion from 2014 to 2017 ($13.6 million per operational day).[37] They planned and prepared for the liberation of Mosul for ten months. They had time and money enough to incorporate coherent medical planning, but they did not.

Additionally, the official estimates numbered close to a million citizens left in Mosul, awaiting liberation. What remained of their homes would likely be destroyed, and no one can live on a battlefield, so it was expected that most of them would try to flee as the fighting got closer. The cartwheel plan allowed for civilian displacement. In addition to the routes in, along which the coalition would fight, there were other spokes – safe corridors mapped out through the assault, along which people could escape, in every direction, away from the fighting, coming out while the military went in. If they could keep going, at the end of the safe corridors, there would be safety and aid in whatever form they most needed it. Although it was an international coalition that was raised to fight ISIS, dealing with the displaced of Mosul was to be an internal matter for the host nation, Iraq. It would be for the Iraqi government to liaise with the humanitarian agencies they expected to find at the end of the corridors. But, somehow, the priority for this aspect of the plan was lost. If it sounds impractical to expect occupation-worn, malnourished, terrified, brutalized civilians in flight to keep to their lane, to slow down for checkpoints and exit the city in an orderly fashion ... well, no one had thought in that much detail. Civilian compliance is difficult enough to ensure, even when it's really well planned and communicated. At Mosul, it was never really a plan at all. It was a Concept of Operations note (ConOps, which sounds more formal and organized when it's an acronym) issued by the Iraqi military, and that's all it was – only ever a concept.[38]

So those were the preconditions for casualties – military and civilian – of Mosul. Cartwheels, safe corridors, dense urban environments – and, for the wounded, almost nothing. There were no medical facilities in nearby cities that could fill the gap, because ISIS occupations on their doorsteps had already drained their personnel and materiel resources for their own civilians to breaking point. There were very few medics left inside Mosul that could be relied on to have survived, let alone to be capable of contributing to a medical response, although they would do their best when the time came. A few foreign medical teams had broken away from humanitarian facilities to give some basic combat casualty-care training to Iraqi military medics and were working desperately to make up the difference, but it was already too late. No one deliberately set out to deny medical help to those likely to need it, and this is not about differing standards or attitudes to the value of human life. The coalition went forward stating its intention to abide by the Geneva Convention, because that was the way of war since 1859 and the beginning of the first age of humanitarianism. But the leader of the coalition, Iraq, the host nation, was not able to comply with the Convention's second protocol (the general protection of the wounded, sick and shipwrecked), or fourth protocol (the general protection of the civilian population against the effects of hostilities). Before any of this started, the Iraqi military medical organization should have become Geneva Convention compliant.[39] It should be a box that is checked every time a military coalition is put together, because no force can be only partly Geneva Convention compliant. It's all or nothing at all. Operation Inherent Resolve was nothing at all, and no one noticed. Hundreds of thousands paid the price of an army going to Mosul with about the same medical capabilities as those at Solferino. Everything Dunant had worked for and created 160 years earlier was gone. Everything changed at Mosul.

Meanwhile, beyond the other end of the spokes on the cartwheel, beyond the huge military force generation camps (which used to be called marshalling or embarkation camps back in the day: the place where resources, capabilities and readiness are assembled at the right scale to accomplish the mission), there were other kinds of planning. There were humanitarian agencies in the region, already strained by the bloody liberations of Ramadi, Tikrit and Fallujah. From all of these places, reduced to mountains of rubble, there were thousands of military and civilian casualties, and tens of thousands of refugees fleeing towards what they hoped was safety, somewhere. Fallujah is a much smaller city than Mosul, and was the first to be fully occupied by ISIS. The mere mention of Fallujah makes humanitarians shudder. As its liberation proceeded, 50,000 citizens fled out into the Anbar desert, towards unfinished, poorly supplied camps. The camps still weren't ready when all the big agencies gathered together again under the UN Office for the Coordination of Humanitarian Affairs (OCHA) and took their collective deep breath to prepare for Mosul.[40]

The start of this kind of humanitarian intervention is the equivalent of the start of any of the world's marathon road races. Hundreds of thousands of people crowd a narrow starting point, pressing forward at any pace they can manage, along a fixed route, until they begin to thin out and speed up, but always keeping going, no matter what their age or state of health or burden, towards the finish line. Mosul would be a marathon, with what the organizers calculated would be at least 800,000 runners, fleeing towards a finish line that had yet to be built. But, in marathons, only one gun ever fires. Not the case at Mosul. In marathons, the principle of support is to keep the runners running, by ensuring any stops they have to make are as short as possible. The organizers have race staff along the route, in high-vis gilets, handing out bottles of water that runners can drink or use to splash the dust of the road out of their eyes; blister plasters, gel sweets for a boost of energy and temporary toilets are all provided – anything and everything, just to keep everyone moving on. In the humanitarian world, the equivalent agency that provides food, water, basic hygiene and basic medical care in units that are light and mobile, run by trained people, so those fleeing war hardly have to stop on their journey, is the World Health Organization

(WHO). Each of their units flies their distinctive light-blue flag, on which the symbol of the United Nations (a polar azimuthal equidistant map of the world, surrounded by two olive branches) is overlaid with the Rod of Asclepius, the symbol of medicine. It is the job of the WHO to maintain the health of the people of the world, wherever it is challenged – something we have all come to understand in much greater detail recently. The WHO at Mosul set out to do its job by planning, supplying and manning the aid posts to maintain the health of those civilians fleeing the city, so they could keep fleeing out of danger and towards safety. For those who reached their aid posts and needed more than just refreshments to keep going, they set up an ambulance service (too informal to be called a corps, and mostly just taxis), and assumed that the transport times could be calculated roughly as average speed x distance (this was perhaps the most naïve assumption they made). In the system designed for Mosul, they had done their part of the job: basic supplies, support, primary healthcare and transportation. The *H* in WHO stands for Health.

At Mosul, the WHO were components in the system, not all of it. It is other international organizations who deal with the serious casualties in conflict zones – the wounded, the extremely pregnant, the very sick, those with traumatic injuries who cannot keep going, who are not strong enough to survive even for a short journey in a proper ambulance. For those who need medical – probably surgical – intervention, right there and then, the traditional, standard provider of trauma care is the International Committee of the Red Cross, usually alongside another INGO, Médecins Sans Frontières. Together, these two organizations had the staff, the mobile trauma units, the kit and the expertise to make up the rest of the medical system that was being set up at Mosul for its fleeing civilian wounded. The ICRC and MSF were already in Iraq, at Ramadi, Tikrit and Fallujah. So, it was assumed – because there was no reason to do otherwise – that they would provide the trauma component at Mosul. If there was a box marked 'confirm civilian refugee trauma care' on the humanitarian planning sheet, it went unticked. In all the meetings in complicated UN/OCHA settings, somehow the actuality of provision was lost, and all that remained were the assumptions. And so, each for their own different set of reasons, both humanitarian and military planning had arrived at almost exactly the same point when it came to Mosul's wounded. They'd assumed that a system was somehow there, and would somehow work, even though it didn't actually exist in reality.

In the middle of all these assumptions, liberation began. On 16 October 2016, the Iraqi and coalition forces headed out from a point forty kilometres from their objective of the al-Nuri mosque. They made quick progress, encircling the city, as they'd planned, ready to make flanking movements into their allocated segments. In liberations, this is always the easy part, so no one gets points for encirclement. Everyone inside the city knew the liberation forces were getting closer, but for all the talk of imminent freedom broadcast in their direction by the Iraqi government, the population of Mosul just tried to stay out of the way. The historian reported on 26 October that, 'Today, Mosul has entered the atmosphere of the war. The bombardment is continuous on many areas of the city, specifically the southern and north-eastern outskirts of the city. Many civilian casualties were reported due to the bombing.'

The historian went on watching, listening, posting constant reports as liberation came closer, dread replacing his earlier exultation. ISIS executed twelve civilians, two days after liberation began. They moved around quickly on motorcycles, especially to the industrial districts, which they had converted into bomb factories, churning out cars and trucks filled with explosives and shrapnel fragments, to be driven at the advancing forces, or buried in the rubble or parked under bridges, so citizens were even more fearful to leave their homes. The historian heard that ISIS called aircraft 'flys', like al-Qaeda had done, which for him meant there were experienced al-Qaeda foot soldiers among them, who had arrived with other foreign fighters, ready for the battle. The historian watched as they fortified key buildings, dug tunnels from which to launch attacks, and installed heavy machine guns and rocket launchers on flat roofs all over the city. He heard that every single bridge across the river was booby-trapped. If he carefully surfed the web, he saw that ISIS had their own WhatsApp groups and blogs and social media that they used to communicate with each other and their allies outside the city, although at least this meant it was in their interests to keep internet provision consistent. ISIS had money in its bank accounts from its commercial activities, and it had been buying drones and adapting them to fly over the coalition forces to check on their progress and take photographs, which could then be used to target artillery fire. The historian heard that the going rate to escape from Mosul to Turkey was $3,000, and people were selling the very last of their possessions to find the money. And, from somewhere, he got the same figure for likely civilian casualties from Mosul as OCHA had presented at their planning meetings: 'Uncertainty of fate is awaiting over one million citizens in Mosul; a fate of uncertainty that swings between displacement and becoming war casualties is what Mosulis fear the most . . . We feel that ISIL is intended to fight a huge battle in Mosul, and there are no signs of it backing up, withdrawing, or fear.'

The historian waited in his room in the darkness and, like the rest of the city, dreaded being in such a place.[41] When he looked up and beyond the minaret, he saw Death hovering over the city, waiting:

> At this moment that is unlike any other moment, when you get caught in the middle, and both life and death are fighting over you, and you're standing there helplessly waiting . . . in a dark tunnel, afraid to move, afraid to stand still, afraid to breathe, afraid to speak, even afraid to stay silent! . . . This war will take a very long time; it will not be over any time soon. I share with you my fears, my pain and my sorrow. I know you have not done anything to deserve to hear them . . . but I don't see any good in staying silent.

By the end of October, the liberators were twenty kilometres from the al-Nuri mosque and al-Hadba minaret. Two more weeks and they had ten kilometres to go. From then on, things became slower, as is always the way with liberations, and more bloody. No matter how well prepared they are, or how great the advantage, liberators lose the upper hand the moment they enter a city. Encircling didn't mean isolating the city, and ISIS had planned for encirclement, building up supplies, digging tunnels, and turning rubble into minefields, filling it with explosives, piling it across roads, trapping civilians in increasingly smaller vectors. They still had lines of communication and supply out beyond the city, and their allies in the city had armed and joined them to fight. ISIS also identified the al-Hadba minaret as the focus for their last-ditch defence. With all sides heading for the same point, either forward or backwards, Mosul became a much more recognizably conventional battle, with an encircling siege, trapped civilians, territory fought for, foothold by bloody foothold, skirmishes becoming continuous combat.[42] Uncomplicated, mappable, traceable, with a river running through it, Mosul was comparable to Stalingrad, or, as the historian saw it:

> How much Mosul today is like Berlin. Berlin was divided by a cement wall, where Mosul is divided by a wall of fire. To the east of it, a door-to-door war is underway, and huge numbers of people are trapped in their homes, breathing gunpowder instead of Oxygen. What's happening there is terrifying. Those who live on the Eastern side [are] thinking to cross over to the Western side, but they are afraid that the battles will chase them there. And those who live on the Western side, they are also thinking of crossing over to the Eastern side, but they fear to come under fire and their move might delay the liberation and lose everything.

Into November, still no progress from the liberators over the river, and the historian began to falter.

The Western bank is still quiet. People are anxious, but hopeful that the advances of operations on the southern front will eventually lead to put an end to all this quietness and marking the beginning of the battles. What they fear the most is the uncertainty with all this. They keep saying 'Liberating Mosul's airport will bring us hope', because they feel the operations on the Eastern bank are taking much longer than anticipated. And ISIS is constantly patrolling the Western bank.

[On t]he Eastern bank, however, people are living a bigger fear; they are constantly under fire, ISIS is bombing the heavily occupied residential areas with mortar shells and people are stranded inside their homes, don't know what to do, or where to go!

Liberation was slowing almost to failure. The rate of gains went from being measured in kilometres per day to single-figure metres. A century after the Battle of the Somme on Europe's Western Front, Mosul had an almost identical rate-of-gain metric and its own no man's land. The area around Mosul was full of casualties – wounded, as one Mosul doctor would later remember, from head to toe[43] – but empty of the trauma care providers that OCHA and the WHO had expected to be there, who they assumed were there already, gloved and masked and working in the worst of it. MSF had been there briefly, but the conditions were too dangerous for their staff, and there was no ICRC trauma team presence either. So, no one was there, and, just as at Solferino, there was nothing but unceasing cries from the wounded, near and far. In response, through OCHA, came an urgent, desperate request from the WHO – the only organization

close enough to hear the cries of the wounded from their aid posts
– to the organizations that they had been dealing with for decades,
asking them to fill the gaps. And this was the moment when the
International Committee of the Red Cross, who had chosen not
to exercise their right of initiative before liberation began, formally
declined to come to the battlefield. The WHO were on their own.

There was no time to argue the case. No time for analysis, no time
to call another meeting and ask why. There was no one else on the
ground. By default, the WHO became the last resort. Default at the
UN is an official process (thank goodness), so it is more accurate
to write that, as per their mandate, the WHO became the Provider
of Last Resort (PoLR). We've forgotten, or perhaps we never knew,
about the PoLR mandate. The last resort in times of particular crisis
– when human beings are in physical danger, when no one can think
of anyone else – is the World Health Organization. Before Mosul, the
PoLR mandate meant sending WHO teams very quickly to relatively
small-scale events that needed primary-care management. They had
just started putting together some trauma capability of their own, but
they were still drawing up emergency trauma-provision standards
and recruiting personnel, so their teams were small, inexperienced
in working together, and in the wrong parts of the world. What they
had wasn't enough. Where they had expected presence, there was
only ICRC absence, and there was no local or military resource to
draw on.

So here, at the point of last resort, the WHO held a meeting
with all their emergency-team staff and asked them to reach out to
everyone in the humanitarian world and beyond, to beg them to

please come to Mosul, come as close as they could, to whatever place they felt the risk to themselves and their staff was acceptable. Come into no man's land and help the people who can get no further. The answer to their call came in a very different way from what they had been expecting. The hands that went up, from the organizations that were prepared to be counted, were all commercial humanitarian groups. The first three were small existing NGOs: NYC Medics, Aspen Medical and Samaritan's Purse (more about each of them later). They aren't charities, although they accept donations, and they don't receive direct funding from governments or US agencies. It's also important to note that they aren't in it for the money. They seek to generate enough funding so their staff can keep going to emergencies and provide support. That's their financial model: they charge for their time and their services, and they bring their own supplies. Up until December 2016, all of their chargeable time had been spent providing backup to the main humanitarian agencies at natural disasters like earthquakes or tsunamis. None of these organizations had ever officially been to war before, although plenty of their employees had. Most were staffed by experienced emergency medical technicians, nurses and surgeons, many of whom were former military medics who had been to Iraq and Afghanistan in a different official capacity, and were very experienced in battlefield casualty. They were an entirely new resource for the WHO to send into the no man's land around Mosul – entirely new, and all they had.

So emails with huge attachments were sent around the world to arrange for this new resource to get to work: contracts, and due diligence, and insurance, and visas. Groups had to change their status so they were officially NGOs, or subcontract to other groups who were already contracting directly with the WHO. They had to be sent to the places where the need was greatest, and hope that there was someone they could liaise with when they finally arrived. They had to find somewhere to sleep, to stow their stuff, to work out from maps and the locals where the roads were and what direction the fighting was in. They needed somewhere to charge their phones. The WHO asked them to plug three specific gaps in the medical system, and they based their request on what they already knew worked in the standard military medical process. They needed trauma stabilization points, where patients stay for twenty minutes while their lives are immediately saved. They needed field hospitals, hopefully not too far away from the stabilization points, where patients stay for up to forty-eight hours and have some damage-control surgery. And they needed more proper hospitals, either existing, reopened or refurbished, where patients stay for however long is necessary, until they can be discharged back to whatever their lives have become in the meantime. All of these would preferably be inside Nineveh province. Beyond Nineveh province was the territory designated the Kurdish Governorate, and crossing the border between them was complicated, took far too long and usually required a change of vehicle.

And while those conversations were being had, the WHO also had to explain – emphasizing rigorously to their new contractees – that they must all, no matter what, do the preprinted WHO patient paperwork, so that case details, dates of injury, treatment and what is required next could accompany the patient on the move through the system. Without paperwork, the system could never be a system, and no analytics would ever be possible, if someone was ever to get around to doing them in the future. Finally, they must all send someone to the regular WHO liaison meetings in Erbil. Erbil, as the capital of the Kurdish Governorate, was almost another country, so they also had to allow enough time to make the border crossing and change vehicles, and, if it took them hours to get there, so be it. These meetings, along with casualty records, meant there could be some sense of what was really happening on the ground, day by day – some sense of what being a Provider of Last Resort really looked like.

And so, at Mosul, from November 2017, as liberation grew ever bloodier, the WHO managed to cobble together a coalition of their own to provide a humanitarian medical response unlike any other assembled in human history. Eventually, there would be seventeen of the contracted commercial NGOs in what is now termed 'a coalition of non-traditional humanitarian partners'. Whatever the official term, the places and systems they set up constitute the first identifiable infrastructure of the second age of humanitarianism.

The non-traditional coalition partners that I know best are those from Global Response Management (who were subcontracted to NYC Medics). GRM's primary capability is to provide emergency care for the severely wounded, and they are as good at it as anyone or any group on the planet. At Mosul, its main players were Pete Reed (a former Marine Corps infantry medic), Alex Potter (a civilian EMT nurse, who speaks the most proficient Arabic of the group) and Helen Perry (who spent five years on active service as a nurse in the US army). Pete was one of those who'd taken himself to Iraq for two years before the liberation of Mosul began, moving around, training small groups of Kurdish military medics to prepare for the inevitable assault. He'd worked alongside medics who had escaped from Mosul but wanted to continue to help their fellow Mosulis when the time came. So GRM personnel already knew the terrain, and had learned how to quickly find a good site for their aid post, how to repair power and water sources, how to find the person who had the latest and best intelligence, especially about transport and what roads were open, what checkpoints worked best and where there were likely to be stashes of supplies, especially antibiotics.

As per their coalition remit from the WHO, GRM hit the battle-ground running, and set up trauma stabilization posts, which they described to me as being 'rough and ready, like MacGyver'. They told me they had learned (from experience, and partly from Helen reading guidance originally written by Florence Nightingale) that their aid post should ideally be in an actual building, with some kind of solid walls for protection, and that wards should be laid out with patients, hopefully on gurneys or beds, around a central table, so the supplies were in easy reach. If they could, they put the younger patients at the front and the older at the back of the post, and treated the less infected ones first, because the younger, less infected patients had more chance of survival. When the wounded came in, their priority was 'super aggressive haemorrhage control', then pack wounds and start a line of fluids to control shock. They learned that they could do all of this very quickly, and fill in a one-page chart that they'd designed to be simpler than the WHO version they had been allocated, but that did the job just as well and faster. Helen paused at that point to tell me that paperwork is important for reasons beyond administration. Anyone working at a trauma stabilization point wouldn't be able to do that work for very long if they thought there was nothing beyond them, as if they were sending their patients out into a void. In this way, the sight of a sheet of paper clutched tightly in a living patient's bloody hand, ready to be passed on to the next link in the chain, is something really hopeful. This was particularly true as they had to wait so long for the ambulances, which sometimes carried as many as eight patients, for as long as seven hours, with multiple stops for checkpoints, where they would have to unload very sick people, reloading them once they had been given the all-clear by whoever was on guard. They learned that, if they gave the ambulance drivers a small amount of training, they could actually manage the patients they carried and turn transport into something like casualty evacuation.

In December, back on the assault front, metres of progress into the city had turned into no progress at all. The stalemate was rebranded as 'an operational pause to regenerate combat power'.[44] Units moved up to replace the losses of the first phase of the campaign. Thousands of Iraqi military casualties had fallen, and their loss was costly – they had been some of the best and most experienced troops, used too early in the campaign. Ammunition was resupplied and vehicles mended, as thousands of axles had been smashed from the relentless pounding on what passed for roads around the outskirts of the city. The military coalition had taken about a quarter of eastern Mosul so far, with much more to go. Across the rubble and the river, their enemy hunkered down in the narrow streets of the Old City, at home in the wreckage, fighting fast or fighting slow, but always fighting.

In the pause, which was never really a pause because ISIS kept up their brutality, the civilian population started to run; for many, their fear had become overwhelming and they now believed that whatever lay out there had to be safer than what was in the city. They fled, not along safe corridors, because those had only ever been conceptual, but along any way out they could find or scramble over, regardless of buried bombs and sniper fire. They fled as fast as they could on the very few roads still open and clear enough for vehicles, on the tanks of petrol they had been saving for that final day, squeezing people into every last millimetre of space in both back and front seats, sometimes so the doors wouldn't close, even though everyone was aware that moving cars were a target for both sides. They fled, driving somewhere, anywhere, as long as it was out of the city. The flight from Mosul laid down some terrible memories for its children. One twelve-year-old girl recalled that her family got up from a meal they were in the middle of eating: 'we were all very afraid and fled away, with nothing in our hands because a bomb exploded right beside us, even though we didn't know where to go.' And, in December, the historian finally fled the city too, leaving behind less visible friends who carried on his work, crossing the river while he still could in some safety, because ISIS had declared that trying to cross the river was a crime punishable by instant death, with executions held on its banks then and there.

By January 2017, the operational pause was over. Force had been regenerated on both sides of the river, and the liberators moved off; behind them, in their wake, the casualties rolled in. By the end of the month, all of the city on the east bank of the river was in Iraqi hands – late, but back on track. Then, all human and digital-video eyes turned to the Old City and the strong vertical line on the horizon, with its seven decorative bands of brickwork, still standing: the Hunchback minaret. A second pause gave time for the liberators to prepare for Phase Three: Western Mosul. All the while, more non-traditional humanitarian organizations were signing their WHO contracts and making the journey from Baghdad towards the military coalition forces, to reinforce the medical system. Everyone learned as fast as they could, went to the meetings in Erbil and did their paperwork. What military medics call a trauma referral system, which should have been there from the outset, was now keeping pace with the fighting and operating across the battlefield.

The historian had made it through and found somewhere to set up his laptop, and he now felt safe enough to introduce himself to his readers. Dr Omar Mohammed, a teacher at Mosul University, wrote on his blog that, when he'd said goodbye to his family, his mum had hugged him and said she had known he was up to something. From just beyond the lines of the liberation coalition, he continued to watch and report. With every modular bridge unit that he saw heading towards the wide river to make crossing places for the coalition troops, he feared what lay ahead. So he laid out his own historian's doctrine and battle plan:

Mosul MUST BE PROTECTED

All airstrikes and artillery bombing of the old neighbourhoods of Mosul MUST be stopped, and refrain from using heavy artillery to respond to ISIS's fire. ISIS's fire can be treated without the use of heavy artillery.

Al-Hadba minaret has endured severe damages due to the use of heavy artillery fire, and it may collapse at any moment. This minaret is the last standing sign of Mosul's existence.

We urge the international community, the Iraqi military and government to refrain from fighting in the vicinity of the minaret or close to it.

Refrain from targeting the civilians in this battle. The number of civilian casualties in the battle for the Western banks is rising to hundreds, in addition to the thousands of IDPs [internally displaced persons] and war escapees. The main goal of this battle is to protect the civilians therefore, we ask all factions to respect the lives of the civilians and refrain from targeting them.

On 19 February 2017, the liberation of the western bank began. No one would refrain from anything. For Global Response Management, this would be the very worst day of the entire campaign. Their trauma stabilization point had treated 132 badly injured casualties, military and civilian, by nightfall. When Pete Reed remembered, he went quiet and just said, 'Madness.' And the madness went on into the next day and the next. So much work. When Iraqi coalition forces reached what was left of the Old City on the western bank, they crawled their way along the streets, channelled into the narrow alleyways, at risk from torn high-voltage lines, fires, debris clattering down on them and dust inhalation. They were restricted by poor communications and had very little ability to evacuate casualties, even if there were trauma stabilization points as near as they could possibly be. Explosions pounded the city – from the coalition forces, to clear the way ahead, but also from the ISIS booby traps that were everywhere – and a new acronym was born: 'VBIED', the Vehicle-Borne Improvised Explosive Device. All those new cars belonging to ISIS were now being repurposed, packed to every last inch with explosives and shrapnel, driven to where the coalition forces were breaking through and then exploded, their drivers darting away through the tunnel network they had dug under the city. Those civilians that couldn't flee hid in their basements with the remains of their supplies, many made permanently deaf from the shattering, constant pounding of explosions all around them.

Tracking the liberation forces were GRM and the other non-traditional WHO coalition partners as they moved through a series of trauma stabilization aid posts towards and eventually into the Old City. From wherever they worked, the battle was brutal. They learned the VBIED acronym very quickly. What it really meant was huge fragments of everything from glass to thick rubber tyres to twisted metal and petrochemicals blown into a minimum of eighteen casualties per explosion, all the survivors arriving at their post at the same time. Such a variety of injuries inflicted simultaneously could be, when they thought about it later on, 'super interesting'. Anyone that worked as part of the Mosul humanitarian coalition learned the sound of incoming patients making it to their part of the system: a heavy vehicle approaching the aid post at speed, slamming on the brakes, and then all the patients that could be fitted inside almost tipped out – civilian, military, adults and children – and it was for the medics to rush forward, grab their headlamps if it was night-time, and get them inside, on gurneys and assessed, so their journey to the next, safer stage of their treatment could begin. Apart from the military casualties, most of the civilians would be malnourished, so they learned to re-feed the small children quickly and carefully with fluids (but not milk, because milk can cause re-feeding syndrome, where a hugely stressed metabolism goes so far out of balance, it is often fatal. 'Not milk' is an unexpectedly important phrase at a trauma stabilization point).

There were regular meetings at the WHO office in Erbil with all the other non-traditional members of the coalition. All of the coalition members could tell who was based where and doing what because some people came to the meeting in clean office clothes, while others arrived in the dusty bloodstained scrub/hiking gear combination that is the uniform of emergency medics on the rough and ready front line. One of the other providers was Aspen Medical, from Australia, who would eventually run three hospitals providing primarily obstetric care, because no one wanted to have their baby in Mosul, but they waited until the last possible moment to make a run for it (obstetric care in the city was very poor and many of the babies were born small). Another provider, Samaritan's Purse, ran a substantial and effective field hospital, with their own security, and brought in a plane with their own supplies. They even had special dispensation to bring in narcotics so there would be strong medication for human beings suffering their way through painful injuries and treatment. It was good for all the non-traditional members of the coalition to meet each other and talk, beyond the official WHO-hosted meeting, even if it meant being away from their own trauma posts, because they could check each other's mobile numbers and contact details. The trauma referral pathway, from stabilization post to field hospital to proper hospital, took a long while to work, and being able to call ahead to someone they knew, to give the numbers of sick and the ambulances to expect, was helpful.

Although their coalition was holding, the WHO was beginning to realize its complications. Some of their partners were really very non-traditional. Samaritan's Purse was among several that provided medical care within a non-denominational evangelical context – 'helping in Jesus' name'. Like Global Response Management, they'd been in Iraq for a while before Mosul, so they knew what to expect and they got on the front foot quickly and stayed there. Samaritan's Purse is well funded by its supporters, and, like all the non-traditional partners, they paid local staff well, better than the going rate, but traditional NGOs say they skewed the marketplace. As it turned out, issues of faith were never really a problem. By far the biggest complication came from the non-traditional coalition members' relationship with the various components of the military coalition. There were small things, like wearing Iraqi uniform jackets that they had been given by grateful soldiers whose comrades they had treated, rather than the scrub/hiking combination that marked them out more clearly as medics. And there were big things, really big things, which will determine what the second age of humanitarianism will be – like being co-located with members of the Iraqi military coalition, and being dependent on them for security, which is the very opposite of neutrality as defined by the International Committee of the Red Cross from their starting point at Solferino.

The non-traditional members of the WHO's coalition weren't naïve or concerned about co-location. It was the precondition to their participation. Co-locating with the military meant they could get to within 800 metres of the front line, and their staff would be protected as far as possible. So the WHO coalition existed within the military coalition, which the WHO could tolerate as the Provider of Last Resort, and the non-traditional partners didn't even have to think about, because they were, as Alex from Global Response Management put it, 'transparently not neutral'. And it wasn't just a question of being within Iraq military units as separate entities. Non-traditional providers actively sought to cooperate with their hosts – to 'bond' with them. They secured their trust by treating their wounded, and more besides. When Iraqi military dead were brought to the aid posts, because their comrades simply didn't know what else to do with them, the providers tended to them too. They took this task seriously, treating them as if they had time, cleaning wounds, arranging them carefully back into a body bag, so they too could make the next stage of their journey. In return, when injured children came through their trauma posts with 'foreign parents deceased' marked on their casualty card, who everyone knew were the children of ISIS, the non-traditional providers asked that they be treated like all the other children and moved along the trauma referral pathway unhindered, and, as far as Global Response Management knew, they were.

Injured adult ISIS fighters remained first and foremost a military problem. Non-traditional medics kept their heads down while Iraqi security officers moved around the medical system, looking to see who might have slipped through and removing them to somewhere else. There were more and more, because liberation had entered its final phase. One of the factors making the difference was the military bulldozers, which were proving to be worth their considerable weight in gold. Armoured bulldozers play well with others, especially combined arms formations, and were surprisingly effective in 'assembling a protective capability in hasty defence' (they are bulletproof and people can hide behind them). They punched through rubble, their drivers became experts at bumping them over uneven ground ahead of troops to clear their way, and ISIS hated them more than anything and targeted them relentlessly. Alex of GRM remembers treating wounded bulldozer drivers and that 'they were awesome'. Or, as they put it in military speak: 'In Mosul, heavy engineer platforms were vital and created a significant conundrum for the adversary.'[45]

The final phase began at a level of intensity no one thought possible. Eighty-five per cent of all liberation coalition casualties would be inflicted in this period. There was nowhere that ISIS did not fight, not a stone left unturned or unshattered. Non-traditional medical teams drove with their military units into the city to help with casualty evacuation, returning to their aid post in the desert at night, to sleep in relative safety, stretched out with exhaustion. They dealt with more and more Mosulis, and it was helpful that there were women medics to deal with women casualties in small improvised private, respectful spaces. On 21 June 2017, coalition troops fought less than fifty metres away from the al-Nuri mosque, in one of the last pitched battles with the occupiers. It was one explosion among many, but when the eyes of Mosul turned to the sky as the smoke cleared, the last standing symbol of the city, the al-Hadba minaret, was gone. A millennium's worth of resilience and seven bands of decorative brickwork had been smashed, the empty sky confirmed by a satellite overpass a day later. The offensive and defensive objective of both sides was, in the end, destroyed by ISIS as they made their last stand. The Global Response Management team never saw the minaret for themselves, but they opened a medical aid post in a convenience store in a building next to the remains of the mosque, an echo back almost a thousand years to the hospital Ibn Jubayr had marvelled at in almost exactly the same place. On 10 July, it was announced that liberation was complete.

Soon after, a fleet of armoured vehicles could be seen making its way carefully and discreetly into parts of the Old City deemed safe enough. There were many convoys finding their way through Mosul in those chaotic days, but this was something else. On board were several research teams, brought together during the years of occupation and commissioned by an international group of universities and humanitarian health institutions to gather data so that the world could have a properly scientific statistical sense of what happened there and what liberation really means. The teams trained in Baghdad, creating a set list of questions that could be asked quickly about some of the most basic facts of life and survival. Each was made up of three women and one man, all medics with doctorates in community medicine (the branch of medicine dealing with healthcare issues affecting communities as a whole). They identified 1,200 households (containing 7,559 people), all of which had been continuously (miraculously) present in Mosul since the very first day of occupation. Using rigorous statistical methodology, the households had been chosen through a 'two-stage 40-cluster survey' – randomly, and evenly spread either side of the river.[46] All of it was easier said than done. When they arrived, each team received permission from the head of the household to undertake the interview, but their primary informant was always the most senior woman. The interviews were quick, about an hour, and took place in conditions of absolute privacy and safety for both sides – probably in the basement rooms that had somehow sheltered the families. If they were able, the teams then went next door, to the right, if the building was still there, and asked the same questions about living conditions, health needs, injuries and deaths. To avoid drawing attention to themselves, they moved 'cautiously' between buildings and conducted most of their interviews in the middle of the day, when there were fewer people about. They kept in constant contact with their supervisors, and they identified emergency shelter locations to which they could flee, should they need protection. Then they went back to Baghdad and wrote up their findings with colleagues from outside Iraq, who were profoundly appreciative of their bravery, and their physical and emotional stamina.

They have kept going back. A second group, comprising medical doctors from Mosul who had fled ahead of ISIS, went in to speak to healthcare workers who had stayed in the city to try to make something like a healthcare system work. Again, these healthcare workers were mostly (but not exclusively) women, mostly married, mostly physicians – the first medical workers from Mosul to be asked about their experiences in this way. From them, the researchers learned that, of all the pressures, the worst was the constant monitoring by the Hesba police, that, every moment of every day, they worked against their will and lived in utter dread, from the moment the black flag was hoisted above the Hunchback minaret, until the final explosions that brought them both down.[47] Their reports and analytics have become known collectively as the 'Mosul Death and Injuries Study' and they have been published in academic journals and on open-access humanitarian data-exchange platforms, with graphs and tables. This was sound, scrupulous scientific methodology, in circumstances where any kind of science had seemed almost impossible.[48] Good reports, clearly and bravely written, hold a very strong part of the line against the Horsemen, even when it's hardest of all to do, as when the team went to speak to the Yazidi households, those few that had survived, in refugee camps. The phrase 'Died on Mount Sinjar' – their mountain, as the historian had described it in his testimony from the time – became a repeating variable on their graph axis labels.[49]

Much of what they found echoed the historian's observations. They tracked the price of cooking gas, and vegetables, and confirmed the destruction of the water purification facilities. They gave numbers for the children held back from school, and they also noted that they saw schools reopening, with volunteer teachers, and parents, with the explosions still ringing in their ears, clambering over rubble to get their children somewhere their education could recommence. Above all, they found that mortality and injury rates were much higher during the nine months of liberation than they had been during the entire twenty-nine months of exclusive ISIS occupation, and the need for trauma care was greater than had been assumed or imagined. They provided statistical confirmation that liberation is always the bloodiest part of war. Of the reported non-intentional, non-violent deaths, they found that cardiovascular disease was, unsurprisingly, the most prevalent, and that domestic violence was also much higher than the norm. Both were signs of the extreme stress of living in the city, and the team noted that these stresses will almost certainly continue in what 'will be a difficult and prolonged recovery of the city'. As they drove away, it was through increasingly large groups of people, carrying belongings – a sign that the city's population had started to come home to Mosul. It was extremely dangerous to return – at least fifteen people were killed on one of the first days of liberation, trying to retrieve belongings from their booby-trapped houses. The first priority for everyone returning to or emerging from their homes, and who was strong enough, was the clearing of the dead. The memory of many who went into Mosul at that time is not so much of the rubble and destruction, but of the smell and the flies.

The UN environment agency calculated that, after liberation, there were eleven million tonnes of rubble in Mosul's streets, most of it on the western bank (the memorable statistic all their press officers cite is that this is the equivalent of three Great Pyramids of Giza). Since July 2017, trucks bearing it away have trundled in and out of the city, day and night (on dirty polluting engines). Some is to be recycled in other buildings, and the flashes of Nineveh's ancient marble show how using the ruined old city to build a new one has been going on all over again. It's still not safe (IEDs continue to be unearthed and diffused) and they haven't found all the bodies, so despite the best, most careful work by the university team, we don't know how many people were killed during occupation and liberation, and we may never know. Current UN thinking is that it will take $90 billion and at least ten years to rebuild the city.

The historian now reports on the rebirth of the city, with the same eye for detail that he had for its destruction. One of the first things he did after he came home was to organize musicians to play Mozart, just as he dreamed, on a warm summer evening, in an informal concert of violins and clarinets. They played under a topaz blue sky, empty of minaret, but at least there was music in the city once again. He's photographed the markets reopening, farmers in the surrounding areas getting back to their land ('markers of normality' in UN-speak), students returning and graduating from the university. He reports on the ongoing catastrophes, smaller in scale, but still about death and waste. In March 2019, Mosulis went to the banks of the river and its

islands to celebrate Mother's Day and New Year (Nowruz). The
weather was spring perfect and there were picnics for larus birds
to swoop on and games for whole families to play. Three hundred
people had crammed on to a ferry to cross the river to one of the
islands that had a funfair on it – except it wasn't a ferry, it was a
portion of a military floating bridge left behind after liberation,
never intended to be a ferry, there to provide crossing points until
the main bridges were rebuilt. Weighted down by too many passengers, crossing a river in high water from spring rains, the unit
overturned, drowning over a hundred people, mostly mothers
and children, their bodies swept away, never to be found, war
or peace. No one comes out of it well: not the medical system,
whose response was slow and inadequate; not the river police and
fire brigade, who had no water search-and-retrieval training; and
certainly not the military helicopter, which hovered over the water,
its downdraft making everything worse.

Elsewhere, and ongoing, there is a growing understanding of what
has not quite been lost forever. Despite the ISIS winter, Mosuli
agriculture has not been mortally wounded. The UN's Food and
Agriculture Organization (FAO) is as committed as UNESCO to
restoring its structure. There's talk of investigating where ancient
irrigation canals were dug from the Tigris to the fields and groves
of the valley, because most ancient canal builders really knew what
they were doing. All kinds of crops are being grown and traded again,
including pistachio-nut trees, which are being replanted in the hope
of reviving the exports that flourished for centuries, providing all the
neighbouring countries with their favourite snack. The soap market

has reopened. Soap is never just a domestic detail. The Aleppo process, which uses olive oil, laurel bay-leaf extract and an alkali derived
from samphire in its ancient recipe, takes nine months and some very
complicated chemical work before the product is properly cured.[50]
Which means soap makers have to judge that there are likely to be
at least as many months of stability from the moment they measure
out the expensive ingredients into their saponification cauldrons and
sweep the stone cellars where the hand-cut cubes will be matured.
Women are back working in Mosul's clothing factories, using their
sewing-machine skills to make garments again – although, from
April 2020, they set aside their dress and shirt patterns to make
personal protective equipment and face masks for the network of
pharmacies and government agencies who needed them during the
COVID pandemic. The historian has learned to write his name in
Yazidi.

Everyone in Mosul knows what would make things eternally
better: to have their Hunchback minaret restored to them, something there when they look up into the sky, something that's simple
and that everyone understands, because Iraqi national politics continues to be difficult and complicated. So, plans – good, solid ones
– have been put into operation to rebuild the mosque and minaret.
UNESCO came back, after the interruption of occupation, and
have brought with them commitment, engagement, management
experience and, above all, enough money. It took them two years to
achieve their coalition of local, central and military authorities, and
the owner of the site itself, and for them to give approval for work
to begin. In November 2019, they finished clearing the rubble from

the site, along with the last of the mines hidden there, because ISIS knew that Mosul would try to rebuild itself, and this was their way of reaching forward from defeat to inflict a few more final deaths. The UNESCO team has made the base of the minaret safe, and this assumes that they'll be rebuilding from it, when it's strong enough, back up into the same piece of sky that Ibn Jubayr saw, centuries before.

The process of exactly how it will be rebuilt will be super interesting. It's not that the minaret couldn't be rebuilt as a hunchback, with its lean clearly visible (that's simply a question for structural engineers, who could use brick and concrete, either shaped or lean-enabling); it's that architects generally don't approve of putting up anything that isn't as it was originally built and conceived. The lean was a flaw, and a new minaret would offer the possibility of correction. Architects love to correct a flaw. But they'll be up against the entire population of Mosul, and history, because, in the consultation exercises done in October 2018 by UNESCO, where they asked experts as well as community groups how they wanted their new minaret to look, the majority said they wanted it the way it was before, with the lean. There's been nothing formally decided yet, but so far it looks like Mosul wants its Hunchback back, just the way they remember it. It's been a very long time since that many Mosulis have agreed about anything, so hopefully, just like the reinforced base of the minaret, that's a consensus strong enough to build on.

'Revive the Spirit of Mosul' is UNESCO's flagship initiative in the region (and its logo incorporates a leaning minaret, so I think it gives a sense of what the final decision will be, although it is still not completely determined). It isn't just about rebuilding the mosque and minaret. They are, as always, symbols of how Mosul itself will be restored, in all its glorious diversity, a mosaic of culture, history and intellectual expression. The money will also be used to rebuild the tomb of Younis and the market at Bab al-Saray in the Old City, known for a thousand years as the centre of both the spice and book trade, where ideas and goods from China and India found their way along the Silk Road, through Mosul and on into Europe. They are stabilizing the foundations of the al-Saa'a Catholic church, which everyone knows in the city, no matter what their faith, because it has a big clock face on its tower and, in the days before phones, it told the time to whoever looked up at it. And UNESCO are rebuilding the Central Library in Mosul University and restocking the books and artefacts destroyed in the occupation, restoring the great repositories of knowledge so nearly vanished.

UNESCO's restoration work is generating jobs, none of which could really be termed unskilled, because rubble and mine clearance needs to be done extremely carefully, by hand, piece by piece, and for a good while longer. Fragments of white marble from ancient ruins can suddenly catch the sunlight through the rubble, and they are carefully dug out and quickly carried away to a work site to be repurposed and recycled, as Mosulis have always done. They'll also need scaffolders, carpenters, metal workers, electricians, painters, engineers and much more. To rebuild the city is also to rebuild the foundation of the city's economy, keeping the extremist wolf from the door of thousands of families, where members are able to work in safety and security, and come home at night, their wages ungarnished. UNESCO is hiring poets and artists and musicians too, because the project is also about restoring the intellectual life of the city that was always so vital. It's not just about replacing the books and opening the bookshops, it's also about reviving book forums and festivals where people can come and argue about literature and its meanings. They are planning artworks and sculpture to go on public view, in the streets, establishing community culture as more than a memory. They are already rebuilding thirty-four houses of the Old City, those that remain, and sometimes, as they dig through the rubble, all the different strands of their work come together. One day, a single stone was uncovered that looked different to all the other wreckage, like something somehow special. A hand in a heavy work glove gently brushed away the dust and debris, and those gathered around managed to read an inscription carved on to the flat surface. It told them that the site they were clearing had been the home of another Mosuli historian (and poet), Yahia al-Jalili, who wrote a beautiful verse and had it put as a keystone on the new house he had built for his family in 1759. The stone bore a message to his descendants who would live after them. There were still traces of the yellow paint used to decorate the stone, and to brighten the walls of a place

> built with blessings and happiness,
> that removed all sadness and protected its heart.
> So my beloved ones, write the history
> That brought life to your house.

And, across the centuries, al-Jalili's message was received, even if, for Omar Mohammed, to write his history of Mosul was to tell of nothing but sadness, and of something very close to death during the occupation. And then, returning to tell a new history, he witnessed how the heart of the city had somehow, almost impossibly, not been broken. He has kept telling its history, despite experiencing a very different kind of *confinement* during the COVID pandemic in 2020, while teaching in France, at the Paris Institute of Political Studies (better known as Sciences Po). And he has continued holding the line, every waking moment of every day, because he cannot really imagine doing anything else. On 22 May 2020, for instance, he wrote, 'I went out walking to get some fresh air in Paris. I found myself in Mosul. This city will never leave me even if I try to leave her.'

Holding a line against the Horsemen in Mosul, making it fast in the oldest city in the world, requires not only a historian to secure our understanding of the past, it needs a new generation to ensure its future. The *E* in UNESCO is for Education. At the heart of the Revive project is the highest-stakes restoration of all: significant investments in access to quality education for the children of Mosul. There is a solid base to start with: parents who understand that schools should be safe spaces – no more terrified teachers or ISIS recruiters prowling at the back of the classroom, no more violent extremism on the curriculum. There are already resources and training for Mosul's teachers, so they can start laying foundations for their students that won't be so easily rocked next time extremists come around, but it's challenging (and there still aren't enough desks and chairs, let alone child psychologists). Their schools are full of displaced and returnee children, boys and girls, of a range of faiths, and they mix with children who grew up or were born under occupation and the last bloody months of liberation, where 'everything was destroyed, and there were dead bodies around and people were crying and bleeding'. (The child who reported this memory of Mosul no longer knew how old she was – twelve or thirteen or fourteen, which would make it difficult for her teacher to know which grade of class would be the correct one for her.) All of them have known nothing but fear for most of their childhood – fear of violence, fear of attacks on them and their families, and constant fear of punishment.[51] When they were asked what was the most frightening thing they remembered, they said ISIS, and bombs, and, very specifically, the dangerous escape from Mosul. And they've all lost someone, or many people, sometimes killed in front of their eyes. Many children experienced domestic violence within their families, either directly or indirectly, just as the mothers of Mosul had told the university team, in private, when they answered the questions for their reports.

Most children from the city have missed years of education, despite their parents desperately trying to make up the difference by home schooling, so, when they eventually go back into a classroom, they can catch up. It's a different kind of catch-up for those who were malnourished, who have growing to do so they can walk to school, and participate in games, and follow the lessons to get back up to the grades they should be getting, so their families can plan for the future. Teachers meet the challenges of students with special needs, with autism and ADHD, as well as the challenges of teaching children who will never quite recover, who'll live with the deep trauma of terror for the rest of their lives, and for whom every step forward is brave. Families and teachers have to find ways to recover profoundly disturbed children who are at the same time perceptive of and hypersensitive to distress. Children who come to school having wet their bed, or exhausted by too little sleep full of 'bad dreams that everything in Mosul is destroyed: the houses, the schools, the people'. They stutter, they bite their nails until they bleed. Of all the childhood conditions reported by parents to the university researchers, behavioural difficulties were the most common, ahead of physical complications. These children will need to learn something as basic as how to play normally, peacefully, to get beyond acting out the dreadful violence to which they were exposed, to go to school as a regular, normal thing. There are children who need to unlearn war and violence and extremism. As one boy (aged ten or twelve, no one was sure) said: 'When I'm angry I want to yell a lot at the person that made me feel angry. Yelling and hitting back makes me feel more relaxed.' That's a hard connection to break. Part of what teachers can do while waiting for resources from central government is to encourage painting and drama and playing musical instruments. There are lots of arts and humanities in the restored curriculum. Every child who arrives for school clutching a breakfast pastry and an exercise book, every face turned towards the teacher in class time, every hand up to answer a question means hope and some healing. Along with their lessons, they are learning how to be children again, and to rediscover joy. But each time a controlled explosion happens, because yet another mine has been discovered in the rubble, or they hear a sudden sharp or shouted word, men arguing, or they see gangs in the playground that get carried away, or sometimes for no obvious reason at all, the children still flinch and cower. Then the work of rebuilding begins again, brick by brick, lesson by lesson, child by child – the real infrastructure of the city.

Everything changed at Mosul. In addition to the first research teams that studied the effects of occupation and liberation on households and healthcare workers, there has been another research group studying the consequences of the WHO's non-traditional coalition. Both originate from the same place: the Center for Humanitarian Health, an academic institute based at Johns Hopkins Bloomberg School of Public Health in Baltimore. The Center, formed in 1998, has chosen a hard road to follow. They work 'for a better future for humanitarian health', and try to achieve it by working across disciplines and without stumbling into silos along the way. I know them from their work on Mosul, where they claimed a kind of right to initiative, one that seeks to initiate research and understanding. It is a commonplace in the humanitarian world that gathering data is very difficult. Whole forests' worth of journal articles are devoted to calling for better data, to lamenting the impossibility of progress without getting sufficient data. But the Center for Humanitarian

Health is used to the hard road, so it didn't just call for data, it went out and got it, and it didn't wait around. The Center paid for the household and healthcare-worker studies itself, and got funding from the US Office of Foreign Disaster Assistance and the European Union for the WHO coalition project. Their 'independent study of the trauma referral pathway', now better known as *The Mosul Trauma Response*, was published February 2018, seven months after the battle had formally ended.

If the WHO's coalition of non-traditional partners is the first physical infrastructure of the second age of humanitarianism, then *The Mosul Death and Injuries Study* and *The Mosul Trauma Response* are its first great texts. *The Mosul Death and Injuries Study* is primarily statistical analysis and interpretation, and its findings, down to their last data byte, are available on public access via the Humanitarian Data Exchange platform. Anyone can use them for their own work. If, for instance, they wanted to draw out all the information that specifically relates to children, they could do that. It's all there. Enough data. Progress is possible. And, although *The Mosul Trauma Response* lacks the poetic flourishes of *A Memory of Solferino*, for a report with subheadings and numbered paragraphs, it is every bit as readable as Dunant's work, and just as compelling. Its authors lay out the background and track the chronology of providing a coalition of last resort. To do so, they talked, respectfully, to all the key players, and, for them, the key players included the non-traditional partners in the coalition. Because they are from the Center for Humanitarian Health, they addressed everything from international humanitarian law (complicated to apply) to the prospects for delivering the rehabilitation of traumatic limb injury in refugee camps (difficult to find).

And, even though they knew they could never be definitive about their conclusions, they still drew them:

> The report finds that the WHO-coordinated efforts helped address critical needs in the provision of trauma care for wounded civilians and saved lives. Approximately 1,500–1,800 lives may have been saved by the collective action of responders, based upon available data of varying quality; of those lives saved, an estimated 600–1,300 were civilians.

Since the report was published, no further analysis of all that data that was generated for the WHO has been undertaken, even though it is somewhere in paper or digital form, waiting to be worked on. *The Mosul Trauma Response* figures are difficult to fathom – is this a good number or a bad number? No one is really sure – but they are all we have. They are a place to start, to hold the line. In addition, the report makes a number of recommendations, mostly about the urgent need to clarify and codify the nature of all the elements of future non-traditional humanitarian-medical coalitions, but also including an item on the responsibilities of governments in dealing with militaries who 'do not or are unable to fulfil their obligations' to care for war-wounded civilians. That particular recommendation was (carefully) supported and supplemented by the US army's own Study Group Report, *What*

Mosul Teaches the Force: 'Mosul operations are a case study for how handling internally displaced persons must be planned early and comprehensively.' And, as well as fighting, 'the US Army should be prepared to execute this resource-intensive task in dense urban environments'.[52]

In the humanitarian world, the vital importance of *The Mosul Trauma Response* lies in its willingness to state that the WHO's coalition of non-traditional partners worked. And this makes things complicated because, along with Mosul's citizens, builders and architects, it means the WHO have their own Hunchback minaret decision to make. Do they correct themselves back to their original design, or do they learn to live and function with their new, unconventional shape? In future, if they become the Providers of Last Resort who cannot quite provide from their own resources, will they once again call on non-traditional partners to fill the gaps? And will we get used to it, so that, in time, we don't think of them any other way? There are some indications that they will. In 2019, before the pandemic, their director general spoke of how the WHO should 'not be afraid of outsourcing some of WHO's core functions'.[53] But let's assume that they remember, and they are not afraid. To make future non-traditional coalitions work, they'll need to streamline the recruitment process for their partners, have the paperwork ready to go at a moment's notice and get organizations pre-approved. They'll have to offer training courses, or something like them, on international humanitarian law and the terms of engagement in neutral spaces, so new partners can be aware of potential complications. Global Response Management weren't quite the right kind of NGO when they answered the call to go to Mosul in 2017, which is why they had to subcontract. But as soon as they came home, Alex modified their operational model, so they are the right kind of NGO now, and have defined their own right to initiative. GRM's right to initiative comes from crowdfunding their costs and recruiting volunteers and going where they think they are needed, as soon as they can get there. And, like all the other non-traditional partners, they understand what they represent: a new kind of humanitarianism – pragmatic, realistic, prepared to take risks (and do the paperwork at the same time), and transparently not neutral. They recognize that they also made everything complicated. They talk to anyone who'll listen about their time in the WHO coalition at Mosul, and they hope that their little medical aid post that worked in what would have been the shadow of the Hunchback minaret is somehow part of the solution.

There have been questions asked of the WHO in our most recent history (more about that in the next chapter, on Pestilence). Some of the important questions that have been lost in the turbulence of the 2020 pandemic are about trauma. Have we relied for too long on assumptions and expectations about the providers of trauma care in catastrophes? Does the Provider of Last Resort need to be able to do it all? In time for the next mass-casualty event, the next Mosul, should the WHO broaden their own mandate to include the provision of trauma care under the *H* for Health? Today's WHO will say that they continue to develop their emergency medical team capability, but that doesn't sound like enough. Perhaps it is not for them alone to give the answer. The International Committee of the Red Cross is formally silent on its refusal to attend the battle at Mosul. When the authors of *The Mosul Trauma Response* went to Geneva and sought their contribution, the ICRC indicated that any assumptions that they would fill the trauma provision gaps at Mosul misrepresented their mandate and historical role.[54] That, to date, is all they have to say on the matter. There is no specific reference to the interaction with the WHO at Mosul in their 2016 Near and Middle East Annual Report.[55] It is a significant gap. Explaining it would be less complicated than perhaps they think. Everyone understands why they could not go to the battlefield at Mosul, why they could not risk their principles or their staff. But we need to hear it from them, because their explanation will also define what comes next, for everyone's sake. And because, as a former director of operations at the organization has said, the ICRC has always 'preferred the dilemmas associated with being present'.[56]

Perhaps the biggest question of all is the one we must ask ourselves. If not the WHO, as first resort or last resort, then who? Who do we want to stand for us in the gaps between violence, suffering and relief? If we aren't able to decide, it's obvious what will happen the next time. Horsemen love gaps. Any kind of gap – in a trauma referral pathway, or in the mandates and legal operations of international humanitarian organizations. Gaps allow the Horsemen to ride on through, single file or together. It is time to close this one, time to herald the new, second age of humanitarianism. Everything must change, because of Mosul.

PESTILENCE

'And behold a white horse: and he that sat upon him had a
bow; and a crown was given unto him and he went forth
conquering and to conquer.'

Revelation 6:2

Recently, it's been hard for us to see any other Horseman but this one. The rider of the white horse is the conqueror we didn't really see coming, who has stormed out from the invisible microbiological world all around us. He carries a bow and a quiver full of deadly arrows, and the one he has selected this time is a virus: COVID-19 (COVID for short). He has other arrows bearing microbes that can invade and infect our bodies' tissue or our environment in ways that do us damage (bacteria, fungi, algae, protozoa), but they differ from viruses in one very distinct way. They can all live and reproduce independently, in colonies or on their own, provided there is food. Viruses cannot live independently because they aren't really alive. Viruses need a host particle, something to hang on to, to incorporate with. They can't do the metabolic processes that life requires on their own, so they tag along with some other actual living thing and borrow from them. The living thing doesn't have to be huge or complex – viruses can live up in our troposphere, attached to molecules in atmospheric gases and aerosols – but without a host, viruses are almost nothing, scraps of protein or DNA or RNA, a bit of biomathematics – unalive, but not necessarily undead.

Before COVID, there was Ebola.

The Ebola virus needs more than an aerosol molecule to live on. It can't survive (unlive) in air. It always needs to be attached to the inside of a living host, preferably a fruit bat. The bat passes it on by biting other fruit bats, or monkeys, or great apes (including us).[57] The Ebola virus makes the living creature its host by attaching on to the cell walls of the body's tiniest blood vessels and spreading from there. As it spreads, it weakens the blood-vessel walls and they start to leak blood. Ebola-host blood vessels are unable to repair themselves as they normally would, by clotting, so blood leaks and the virus spreads, and a simple viral infection quickly turns into a huge assault, everywhere at the same time. And the body reacts in kind, fighting back with the complex biological response known as our inflammatory mechanism, which is designed to save us. The bigger the insult, the bigger the inflammatory response. An inflammatory chemical cascade is started that is supposed to control the bleeding, but instead it's spread around the entire system by the blood that is already breaking through the vessel walls. The inflammatory-mechanism chemicals are supposed to be used sparingly by the body, because they are toxic in high quantities, so, when they are carried where they shouldn't be, they poison the victim from within.

We assume that internal bleeding is the most common sign of Ebola's fatality. But it is the effects of a compromised blood circulation and filtration system going untreated – sepsis, septic shock, nerve damage, organ failure and dehydration – that usually kill its victims. It isn't the virus itself that can be deadly, it's the immune response to it, and a good way to remember this is by considering the bat. Bats appear to have a genetic mutation which means their innate immune systems are super-responsive – not because they react very strongly, but because they react just right. Humans who get Ebola die from their defensive mechanisms going into overdrive, or where their weakened immune system can't mount a defence at all. But bats – thirty species checked so far, all the same – can continually modulate their inflammatory response. It probably has something to do with the metabolic demands of being able to fly where they like, swooping quickly from high, colder, lower-oxygenated altitudes, to lower down, amid the trees, where the air is warm and humid. That's our current hypothesis. Whatever it is, it makes bats the ideal hosts for viruses, which can go on unliving inside their bodies for years, without killing or being killed. No other species on Earth can withstand this.[58]

Ebola gets its name from the first recorded outbreak, in 1976, near the Ebola River in the Democratic Republic of the Congo. (Scientists who discover new, potentially deadly viruses try to name them after rivers because it's thought to be unhelpful to name them after villages or towns.) It's a virus with four different strains, and humans pass it on to each other by direct transmission in blood and body fluids. But for all our fear of its effects, Ebola doesn't have to be fatal. If the effects of compromised blood circulation are treated early, most people who catch it will survive. It's all fairly basic medicine, things we do every day when people get ill. We use intravenous drips to replace the fluids and the electrolytes that an illness is causing someone to lose. Keeping the patient properly hydrated, with the correct fluid balance, stops their organs being damaged and rebuilds their body's ability to process toxins. Because blood circulation is threatened, and therefore the body's ability to get its energy from the oxygen in the blood, we give the patient extra oxygen via a facemask. We regulate disordered blood pressure with medication, and control diarrhoea and vomiting, and we use aspirin for fever. Standard treatments all – and, for Ebola patients, intensely and constantly administered until the infection has disappeared. But we have to do it all very, very carefully, because Ebola is so easily transmitted by the blood and body fluids that are being displaced and replaced all the time during the course of the disease. So Ebola patients are admitted to single isolation bays, and are treated by medical staff that have no direct physical access or contact with them, which makes the fairly basic medicine less basic to actually do. But no less effective: as the *Lancet* reminded everyone in 2019, 'the fact that high-level optimized care appears to improve outcomes needs to be promoted to overcome perceptions that Ebola virus disease is fatal and that patients cannot be cured.'[59]

But there were two years in our very recent history when it didn't feel like that. In 2013, in Guinea, close to the borders of Sierra Leone and Liberia, in West Africa, there was an outbreak of the Ebola virus that was the epidemiological equivalent of the Battle of Solferino.[60]

It began here, with a single case: a two-year-old boy, carried into a medical facility by his family, already dying of Ebola. Quickly, members of his family and then the medical staff who had treated him contracted the virus and died. There were already medical NGOs working in the country – in particular, Médecins Sans Frontières – and they identified that it was not a new or especially virulent strain, but that it was serious. In order to control the outbreak, extra resources would be required that were beyond the existing healthcare systems in the affected countries. MSF set up field hospitals in areas where outbreaks had occurred and prepared for more patients. And they did the absolutely fundamental, essential reporting, by filling out the paperwork and emailing or faxing it off to the relevant office at the provider of first resort in the case of disease epidemics: the World Health Organization.

Unlike dealing with trauma arising from conflict or natural disasters, dealing with disease outbreaks is core business for the WHO. Their remit is to be 'the directing and coordinating authority on international health work'. They lead the global response to epidemics, part of which is to monitor closely the spread of diseases. If there are more cases than there should be, across international borders, they declare a Public Health Emergency of International Concern (PHEIC). This is the declaration that mobilizes the international community to provide a coordinated response to an epidemic, either directly by sending staff and supplies, or indirectly by providing funding. There are no dilemmas for the WHO in being present at an Ebola outbreak. They bring their experience, skill and international coordination mandate to deal with a problem

they have already solved many times, to ensure that a serious outbreak doesn't become a crisis. But not this time. By April 2014,
five months after the first case was reported, the virus had surged
out of control, spreading host by host through the country and
into neighbouring West and Central African states, because the
WHO was absent.

The reason wasn't the gathering storm 5,000 kilometres away in
the Iraqi desert, distracting the WHO and draining its resources, nor
was it the significant political instability in the region of the outbreak
itself. In the first ten months of the Ebola outbreak (from December
2013 to August 2014), the leadership of the WHO did almost
nothing except talk. There were talks at the highest levels in the
WHO HQ in Geneva, about a lack of funding, about poor relations
between them and the national WHO offices in the affected countries, about whether it was even their role to be the first responder
in epidemics. But, to the watching, waiting world outside, it looked
like nothing. Journalists from everywhere converged on the outbreak
areas and did pieces to camera in hazmat suits from outside wretched
field hospitals, blaming (not exclusively, but mostly) public burial
rituals for the spread, speculating on how the virus might arrive in
countries beyond Africa, and asking when the WHO was going to
get there. Other organizations arrived and set up, but without the
coordination that only the WHO could offer, there was a limit,
marked out in human lives, to what they could do. Phrases like
'global biodisaster' were bandied about, and suddenly we could hear
the hoofbeats of the white Horseman growing closer, as hundreds
of deaths became tens of thousands.

The WHO was absent because it had no idea what was actually happening on the ground at the outbreak. Their surveillance systems, which should have been the infrastructure of their first response, were out of date, and their modernization had not been prioritized. Any data sent to them by organizations on the ground went unanalysed and unused. It was not until eight months after the first case that the WHO finally looked at the data it had been sent and declared, in August 2014, that the Ebola outbreak was a Public Health Emergency of International Concern. They also issued a road map for affected nations to follow. Not an actual road map, because about the only thing they had done regarding the Ebola outbreak was to issue travel bans to the affected areas for their staff, but a 'road map' strategy and communication tool (downloadable from the internet), which was supposed to give guidance to states affected by the epidemic. So, more or less, still nothing.

In the meantime, on the ground, the medical NGOs and aid organizations did their uncoordinated best to hold the line in health centres and field hospitals where patients could be diagnosed, isolated, treated, buried or discharged. One health worker remembered making sure that, every time a patient was discharged, the entire staff gathered round and clapped and cheered, and then went back to admitting the new cases.[61] But healthy staff, who got enough sleep and had the energy to clap and cheer, and didn't get infected and die, were becoming increasingly scarce. It wasn't just those attending the dead who were at higher risk from Ebola patients. By the end of the epidemic, deaths among health workers (doctors, nurses and midwives) were significantly higher than those among the general population. Across the affected region, over five hundred precious healthcare workers died during the epidemic. Strained healthcare systems buckled, and maternity provision in particular suffered.[62] More babies and mothers died because there were fewer people who knew how to care for them. Dealing with the virus was taking over entire, already burdened national healthcare systems.

PHEIC or no PHEIC, in the continuing absence of the WHO, it became clear to everyone on the ground that someone else would have to provide both vital treatment infrastructure and coordination. The only organizations with anything like the necessary kit and capability were the very last people any of the humanitarian medical agencies generally wanted to be dealing with – national militaries. It is defence forces of nations who prepare and train regularly to deal with the effects of biowarfare and biohazards, whether in chemical or engineered viral form, and this capability can be deftly adapted to deal with natural pathogenic (pathogen = bringer of disease) hazards. It is the world's military and their military medical services who have the protective kit on standby, and the ability to move fast and get it to wherever it is most needed. Henri Dunant had realized after Solferino in 1859 that he would get nowhere in constructing a humanitarian response to the aftermath of battles without the cooperation of 'the princes of the military world.' In September 2014, despite the PHEIC, those fighting Ebola felt they were in something very like a war that was being lost. So the international president of MSF, Joanne Liu, went to the United Nations General Assembly in New York and spoke not just to the world, but to a very specific, operational part of it.

Many of the Member states represented here today have invested heavily in biological threat response. You have a political and humanitarian responsibility to immediately utilize these capabilities in Ebola-affected countries.

To curb the epidemic, it is imperative that States immediately deploy civilian and military assets with expertise in biohazard containment. I call upon you to dispatch your disaster response teams, backed by the full weight of your logistical capabilities. This should be done in close collaboration with the affected countries.

Without this deployment, we will never get the epidemic under control.[63]

This was no careful first-person account, written in hope, as Dunant's *A Memory of Solferino* had been. It was a speech made in barely concealed rage, and repeated beyond the General Assembly to boards specially convened for the purpose, and in short, forcefully written articles across the world's media. But, just as it had been with Dunant's piece, the timing was right, and the effect was the same. Member states rallied their forces, forming another kind of non-traditional humanitarian partnership, and national militaries became the Providers of Last Resort at the Ebola epidemic – not to enforce quarantines or border controls, or control panicking populations, but to contain the biohazard by helping manage the treatment of patients. They came to scale up field hospitals, install and run the laboratories needed for pathology, provide triage centres for diagnosis, assist in the management of the dead, and fly medics and materiel to wherever they were most needed. There was no time to worry about embedding and co-locating. A humanitarian–military coalition was put together as fast as possible, and was moved to where it needed to be, ready to hit the ground working.

And it did. The epidemic was declared over, more or less (hold that thought), by the end of 2015. According to the official statistics, 28,000 patients had needed intensive medical care and 11,000 lives had been lost to the disease itself, although no one knows the actual figure, because of the overwhelming of the medical facilities and staff, and because being really precise about death rates is a very hard thing to do, no matter who you are. The outbreak left behind a regional population shattered by fear and poisoned by the betrayal of the one global organization that was supposed to save them. Sometimes, when I mention the WHO to my colleagues who were in the humanitarian sector at the time, they frown and say that there is a part of them that still hates that little light-blue flag, because they saw it on too many limousines and not enough ambulances. And although there had never been much risk of Ebola becoming a global biodisaster (and we know what that looks like now), perhaps the apocalyptic language about the sound of hoofbeats was justified, because it was exactly this kind of stark image that brought change where it was most needed, at the heart of the WHO.

There were at least four long reports analysing the WHO's failures in the Ebola epidemic of 2013–15. None of them read with the same urgent clarity as *The Mosul Trauma Response*, but they did at least have the courage to draw some conclusions. Blame was apportioned to the 'non-assertive leadership', dreadful interdepartmental communication, lack of funds and waste of those that they had, and the almost non-existent surveillance of disease outbreaks.[64] Maybe something of the spirit of the organization that had held the line at Mosul was making its way back to HQ in Geneva. Or perhaps it was shame. But, whatever it was, the organization suddenly remembered who and where it was supposed to be. Processes became transparent, people in the organization talked to each other again, but in a good, practical way, not too much. Eventually, an entirely new leadership would be openly elected (previous ballots had been in secret), including a new director general, whom we all recognize today as Dr Tedros.

All the organization's existing research that was relevant to Ebola was brought front and centre. Everything of significance that we learned about the science and genetics of Ebola came from this point. There had been Ebola vaccination research dawdling along in labs, including those of the WHO, before 2014. Then, as one researcher put it, 'development was impressively accelerated under intense media attention'. A vaccine was developed, and, alongside it, WHO guidance for Monitored Emergency Use of Unregistered and Investigational Interventions (MEURI), so it could be used to contain the 2017 outbreak without having to wait for lengthy Phase Three protocols to complete. More vaccines and effective antivirals were ready for a second serious outbreak in 2018. We understand now that the Ebola virus can hang on in unexpected places, like intraocular fluid (not tears, which are the one body fluid which doesn't spread the virus), so we need to keep an eye on patients after hospital discharge and be careful about what we designate as a full recovery. We understand that we aren't likely to stamp Ebola out any time soon (partly because we don't yet fully understand the ecology of the virus in wildlife and the zoonotic process whereby pathogens are transferred from animals to humans), so it is always somewhere, awaiting new hosts. But, in the meantime, we can safely and effectively vaccinate the humans that live alongside the virus. By 2018, in addition to huge WHO civilian programmes, 60,000 healthcare workers had been vaccinated across Central and West African countries – and once vaccinated, always vaccinated, as far as we know.

Sixty thousand vaccinated healthcare workers: that's one of the two key metrics to look at as a measure of the WHO transformation after the catastrophe of 2014. Here's the other one: it took just eighteen hours from the very first report of an Ebola case in the Democratic Republic of the Congo in 2017 for the WHO to get boots and kit on the ground in response. Because, in the meantime, they had created an Early Warning and Response System (EWARS) that reconfigured the disease-surveillance space, and they did it by thinking inside the box. An EWARS box looks like a black plastic wheelie suitcase, only a little more rugged, with bigger clunk-clunk locks. Each EWARS box contains the components to initiate and communicate surveillance of a disease outbreak: sixty mobile phones, two powerful laptops, both with the software and apps that connect back to WHO head offices pre-loaded, and solar chargers for all of them. Each EWARS box can keep a sturdy, steady eye on fifty separate health clinics at once and hundreds of thousands of people. Opening up the EWARS box, distributing the phones and computers, and sending back the information is an essential first response to a disease outbreak. Where Ebola was concerned, it meant the WHO knew what was going on almost as soon as the virus got going, and their epidemiologists, as well as their medical teams, could get to work. In the new focused surveillance space created for the WHO, epidemiologists were able to realize that the more data they had, from sources they had never been able to access before, the better their analysis and modelling of current, and therefore future, disease outbreaks would be. Between then and now, a new science has been created: outbreak analytics – where epidemiology meets the cutting edge of data gathering.

Outbreak analytics gallops as fast as any of the Horsemen (both the Ebola vaccine and the new science of outbreak analytics took just under two years to get from concept to practice). Its progress is best understood via a great theme issue of the scientific journal of the Royal Society, *Philosophical Transactions B*. There is a reason that information isn't in a footnote.[65] The *Philosophical Transactions* was founded in 1665, in London, to serve as the peer-reviewed house journal of the oldest scientific academy in the world. In 1672, the *Phil Trans* (as all academics in scientific institutions know it) published Isaac Newton's very first public expression of his work on optics, in the form of 'a letter . . . containing his new theories on light and colours'. When the Royal Society publishes or speaks, it does so with the heft and responsibility of history at its shoulder. In July 2020, when the UK government clarified its advice on the wearing of face masks in enclosed public spaces to prevent the spread of the COVID virus, it was after a rare public intervention by the president of the Royal Society. So, when the journal of the oldest scientific academy in the world publishes an entire theme issue dedicated to the newest of the data sciences, it means more – much more – than the sum of its parts.

What the theme issue describes to the world is how outbreak analytics seeks to bring together a new and unique range of separate disciplines, all in the service of precisely describing and quantifying epidemics as they happen, so that the public health and treatment response is the best it can be, moment by moment. Outbreak analytics links case data – people who have reported to healthcare units with symptoms – and background data – such as geographical or demographic variabilities – and builds models that connect the two.[66] Eventually, when the outbreak is under control, everything that has been learned to deliver treatment and prevent spread is analysed. Counterfactual models are run to see what other options might work, or work better. New methodologies are constructed to update likely vulnerabilities of populations across the world, so that preparation and – ideally, hopefully – prevention can take place. Using vulnerability as a criterion is something new in infection control, but it's become a standard in outbreak analytics. Test where the line is weak. Reinforce it. Allow for no gaps (because we know who loves a gap). Outbreak analytics is the data-science counter to the Four Horsemen – it's about how things work best together, and how to understand them so we can stop them, when we need to, next time.

That's where we were, the day before, in the old normal: outbreak analytics being done by scientists in centres that have been part of collaborating partnerships with the WHO for several years, many of them having spent the worst and most dangerous of times in the field, holding a line against Ebola, getting a grounding in the reality of very sick humans suffering through an epidemic, beyond the numbers – an experience that never leaves them. They were building an early-warning system against what in 2018 was called Disease X – an unknown but virulent pathogen with pandemic potential.[67] Everyone working in the field was refining and integrating all the elements of their developing data science, and pressing for it to become part of a new, super-smart global pandemic Early Warning and Response System, because, as the editors of the *Phil Trans* theme issue said, 'emerging pathogen epidemics remain a major public health concern'. Then, on 31 December 2019, the first COVID case was reported to the WHO office in China, followed by the genetic identification of the novel coronavirus type, a week later. For the new community doing outbreak analytics work, everything came out of the planning phase and went operational, just as it did for the world's medical staff, in real time, real life. X = COVID-19.

Throughout 2020, the world watched as COVID infections spread, and everyone learned the real meaning of 'global biohazard'. Those who had borne or treated or studied the Ebola outbreak found themselves reminded, every moment of every day, of the endurance required to provide care and understanding on such a scale. The hazmat suits were back – 'Ebola armour', as it was named in the 2014 outbreak – heavy, hard to handle and work in, and above all hot, even the fancy new models with the built-in respirators and cooling systems. Wherever Ebola armour is worn, it can only ever be for a short while before it has to be peeled off, the wearer finding a place to cool down, somewhere they don't have to view everything through a fogged visor plate, where they can shower, rest and gather themselves for the next shift. During the Ebola and COVID outbreaks, health-care workers started using Sharpie pens to write their names on their plastic aprons, so, even if their patients couldn't see them behind their masks or armour, they could at least still call out their names individually, human to otherwise-almost-unrecognisable human. Just as the staff in the Ebola clinics had done a few years before, now the rest of the world's medical staff stopped what they were doing and clapped and cheered as the first patients to recover from COVID-19 were wheeled along the hospital corridors to go home, because a few moments of hope is good for everyone, and then they went back to their armour and their wards. Dr Tedros told the world how he would never forget the images of health workers, where the line they held every day for their COVID patients, working behind pressure-sealed filtering face-piece respirators (FFP3 masks), was left as an imprint on their own faces. These were unexpected signs of a Horseman in our midst: grade one facial pressure injuries – sores and bruises – most commonly inflicted on the cheeks and the bridge of the nose, behind the ears or along the jawline of medical staff who wore their FFP3 masks for much, much longer than the recommended one hour.[68]

By the end of 2020, there were formal recommendations for how to deal with facial pressure injuries (barrier creams, wound dressings, painkillers, modified shift patterns), and WHO emergency protocols first developed for Ebola had been updated so new COVID vacci-nation programmes could be undertaken as quickly and as safely as possible.[69] Those working in outbreak analytics also faced sustained pressure, a different kind of endurance, to model and analyse the complexity of the factors and variables that then produced numbers from which government policy was made – and on which lives depended, all over the world. The core science that was brought out of the Ebola epidemic has been scaled up exponentially, day by day, to account, not for complicated science, but for complicated human societies and their variegations in politics, society, government, economics, as well as geography and demographics. There are whole other categories of vulnerability, uncertainty and shift to be accounted for today and considered for tomorrow, when the outbreak analysis models are reviewed, and counterfactuals run, and the gaps and the weaknesses in the line held against the pestilence of COVID can be identified. Only now do we really understand the complexity and potential of outbreak analytics, and just what will be required of those who go on to prepare for the emergence of the next pathogen epidemic, which they will presumably call Disease Y (and which is likely to be based on an influenza-type virus, because many of the arrows carried by the rider of the white horse are flu-tipped).

It is also from Ebola that we get our understanding of how disease outbreaks end in real time, one day to the next. We know what the end of an Ebola epidemic looks like because the WHO set a metric. If, after forty-two days in a surveilled outbreak area, there are no new cases and no new exposures to possible new cases, then an Ebola epidemic may be declared over. The figure of forty-two days comes from taking the twenty-one-day maximum period of incubation for the virus and doubling it, to be on the safe side. We know the name of the last patient from the 2018 Ebola epidemic in the DRC who was treated in hospital, recovered and was discharged. Forty-six of the people on her contact list had also been monitored, but none developed symptoms. So, having given her consent for it to be made public, on 4 March 2020, Semida Masika went home to the cheering celebrations of the medical staff who cared for her at the unit. Her departure was joyfully filmed on the phones of her family and friends, but with much less attention from the world's press; by then, they all had other things to report on in their own backyards.

And from the old normal, a warning for the new: 'Rigorous surveillance is necessary for high confidence in end-of-outbreak declarations and other infectious diseases.' According to the scientists of outbreak analytics, forty-two days may not be helpful when it comes to setting the metric for other viruses, or even for Ebola itself. Forty-two days assumes a high rate of effective epidemiological surveillance, and, so far, it has only been used within one country. The forty-two days metric may not adequately account for the excellent hiding skills of Ebola virus fragments in intraocular fluid, or possible sexual transmission, or travel between regions by people or animals. Confidence in the end-of-outbreak declaration needs to be maintained, or else it becomes just another press release that no one pays much heed, or, worse, it undermines trust. So it ain't over till it's over, or, as the outbreak analysts put it, providing a good, confident end-of-epidemic figure 'might require elaborations to the underlying model'.[70]

Outbreak analytics can be difficult to get our collective head around (unless we're epidemiologists), but vaccines are something

everyone understands. During 2020, we watched and waited –
sometimes day by day, news bulletin by news bulletin – for a
COVID vaccine to be discovered, to be tested, to be approved by
the regulator and to be distributed, in the first instance, to where
it would do the most good. This wasn't an unfamiliar part of the
line for the world's infectious-disease specialists. Many of them
had been there before, or could clearly see the footprints of their
predecessors who had worked to develop an Ebola vaccination that
went from lab to life-saving in eighteen months. It helps, when you
are given an almost impossible task, to know that someone has done
it before, successfully. It helps, also, to know that other thinking,
necessary beyond the lab and medical journal, has also been done.
We know that multiple research projects should be undertaken at
the same time, and while it isn't a race or a competition, that kind of
background sets a tone that reminds everyone time is of the essence,
if the world is to win. The WHO has spruced up the Monitored
Emergency Use of Unregistered and Investigational Interventions
protocol that it began in 2016 specifically so the Ebola vaccine could
be given as quickly as was practically possible and compassionately
necessary. It's now called the Emergency Use Assessment and
Listing (EUAL).[71] There are national and international equivalents
that have allowed for extraordinary research progress to be translated into public vaccination programmes across the world in less
than a year. Nations who hurried to support populations threatened
by COVID-19 could do their vaccine research knowing that the
global provider of first resort had already used their experience and
existing structures to secure a model that made the really difficult

decisions about ethics, regulation, and how to balance those factors against great, urgent human need. The strong part of the line, built by those who had earlier worked on the Ebola vaccine, held. It's therefore not unreasonable to assume that it has been strengthened further for next time. Hopefully.

Right now, the single greatest threat to the eradication of Ebola wherever its epidemics occur isn't the virus itself or any other viruses, but humans at war. Political instability and violence seriously impair the ability of national or international health systems to give care and protection to those who need it. Localized violence causes displacement, so contact tracing becomes impossible, and vaccination and monitoring networks break down. No matter how hard they tried, or how closely they stuck to the terms negotiated for their coalition with the humanitarian agencies, the arrival of international military biohazard teams in 2015, wearing uniforms under hazmat suits, caused tensions in local communities. For all the concern about the non-traditional humanitarian partnerships at Mosul, the one put together to deal with Ebola was just as problematic in the countries where it operated. It undermined what little humanitarian-based neutrality had been maintained, and from there it was a short step to political factions decrying vaccination as aggression and the medical treatment of Ebola cases as imperialism by other means.

The civilian population of the region continues to live with the problems created by the military–humanitarian coalition. Attacks on medical facilities, no matter whose flag they fly, are common in areas where Ebola hangs around, looking for hosts. Humanitarian agencies will only risk the safety of their staff for so long, and national healthcare systems remain under strain. In 2019, four health workers undertaking vaccination programmes in the Democratic Republic of the Congo were killed, and five others badly injured. Dr Tedros mourned the deaths of these 'first responders' in the fight against Ebola. Accounting for the impact of violence, the metrics of fear and the uncertainties of displacement within existing demographics will indeed need to become part of the elaboration of the outbreak analytics model for Ebola's outbreaks and endings. Forty-two days might sound ominous to the rider of the white horse, but to the rider who brings war and who clears the way for the rest of his company to circle round and keep coming, it's just another number.

A lot has happened between 2013 and 2021. It's been a period during which we've learned a significant amount about viruses, but we're still puzzling the alive/undead conundrum. There were virus ancestors to be found on our planet from the very outset – not life forms then, either, but a process or a mechanism that allowed very simple cells to interact – and, whatever they were, they existed only at the point of interaction. Evolutionary biologists who espouse the progressive theory of viral evolution think that this mechanism of being able to move between cells somehow became a thing – a virus. Those who support the regressive theory think that viruses are less than they originally were – perhaps they were a bacterium that evolved to become so dependent on the cells it interacted with that it could exist in no other form but as what we now recognize as some kind of parasite, only able to survive by clinging on to something actually living. Or viruses may have been there all along, before anything else, as self-replicating units of a mechanism, waiting for cells to evolve so they could use them. Or all of the above might be true, no one really knows. It was pretty murky, back then.[72]

We are much more certain that the first living things to emerge from the prebiotic chemical clutter of our planet in its earliest form were primitive kinds of bacteria.[73] Bacteria meet all the criteria scientists have for describing something as living. They can grow, reproduce, maintain an internal equilibrium of their various components, respond to stimuli, metabolize and evolve. Bacteria got going on all of this activity in states that we now call biofilms – where living things stick to each other and to surfaces – and this isn't theoretical, because we have biofilms in the fossil record. There have been bacterial biofilms on the Earth for two billion years and they are the structural solution to the problem of how to survive on planets in their earliest, most chaotic forms. To make a biofilm, you need some kind of fluid (from evaporation) forming some kind of pool in a chemically energetic landscape (the residue from eruptions).[74] Then you need something that scientists aren't quite sure about yet, but classify as 'pre-alive' – another kind of chemical from an eruption – which comes into contact with the surface of the pool of water and chemicals, making a bubble that doesn't quite burst, changing from something that floats in air into something that floats on fluid. And when it happens time and again, and the bubbles connect and a kind of film forms and it doesn't die, then pre-life becomes bacterial life, definitely alive, and pre-biology becomes microbiology.

And then evolution occurs at pace and scale. Biofilms are a mixing point, where elements merge and don't quite break apart, becoming more than the sum of their parts, something that can grow and change and learn. One of the first lessons the new bacterial biofilms learned was: don't dry out, or at least dry out very slowly, so even though their fluid supply might be affected, they wouldn't be.[75] Second lesson: waste nothing. Biofilm bacteria ate and recycled everything around them, in the air or in the fluid, including the pre-alive things. From them, eventually, life in other forms developed – but as an offshoot, not a replacement. Once bacteria found their place, they stayed. So the origins of life aren't exactly a primordial soup, they are the bubbles on the surface of the primordial soup. It's an analytically intractable mixture (the technical scientific term for a mess). Until recently, it put scientists off when they were looking for answers to the where-did-we-come-from question. But now we're getting better at framing an answer, thanks to biofilm bacteria fossils: we came from somewhere hot, where there's water evaporating and there's a chemical mess. And now we know what to look for when we want to see if anyone else is likely to be coming from somewhere – on Mars, for instance. In the Gale Crater on the red planet, there is evidence of hydrological perturbation: evaporation of what was recognisably some kind of water from a lake, leaving behind a range of sulphates and clays, which dry out in a layer of deposition. Then, when the water comes back, even if it's just a few puddles' worth, it has a slightly different chemical composition, and maybe, just maybe, some tenacious-looking bubbles. Earth's latest Mars exploration vehicle, the Perseverance Rover, has been sent to the Jezero Crater, which is the site of an ancient river delta, because that also looks promising for a microbiological fossil hunt.[76] And it's not just Mars. There are trace gases in the cloud decks of Venus that may have been generated by some kind of bacteria.[77] Titan, the largest of Saturn's moons, has an atmosphere that is similar to an early Earth. We know where that might lead, eventually.[78]

Bacteria are able to live anywhere you can think of, inside and outside other living creatures, as long as there's food so they can survive and reproduce. Bacterial ecologists have a motto about the subject of their study: 'everything gets everywhere'.[79] Today's microbiologists can't tell you anything about bacterial biofilms that evolutionary microbiologists don't already know, and they all agree that 'biofilms are one of the most widely distributed and successful modes of life on earth'.[80] They are much better at living than we are. Biofilms are an organized cluster – a matrix – of short, round bacteria, which is very strong and very sticky. They are non-motile, so they move the same way they grow, by reproducing and increasing their surface area.

The more today's microbiologists look at biofilms, the more they (and we) are amazed and fearful of their abilities. Biofilms are able to use electrochemical signalling to pass messages around their community. Those who live on the outside of the biofilm do most of the eating, so they tend to be bigger than those in the interior. When the difference between interior and exterior becomes unmanageable, a signal is sent out to stop consumption at the edge and let the nutrients spread through the cells until a balance is restored. The same thing happens if the biofilm needs to defend itself. If the exterior cells are destroyed by something like, say, an antibiotic chemical, then they can die and quickly be replaced by fit interior cells, up for a whole new fight. We can see the signalling as it happens (with a good enough microscope), as the messages are fired around the community like tiny bolts of coloured lightning. They aren't supposed to be able to do this, because they don't have the right kinds of cells for communication, but it turns out they can do it anyway.

The world belonged to bacteria, aeons before other living things evolved, before the idea of the Horsemen, and it may be that bacteria have taken a long hard look at things since humans took over, and perhaps they think, all things considered, they'd like the planet back. The signalling research findings prove that some bacteria can talk among themselves, and it would be useful for us to understand things like how much of this language bacteria already speak from way back when, and how quickly they can learn new forms of communication when reacting to a change of circumstance.[81] Because, between the prebiotic soup and the human today, at some point a white horse rode by, and the rider leaned down and picked up a new set of weapons so he could go forth and conquer as Pestilence.[82]

Bacteria prosper when humans don't. When we get diseases or wounds, or we're starving, when all these things impact the cells in our tissue, the balance of power shifts and bacteria move in, taking our remaining energy for their own. Over the centuries, they've found the easiest pickings when humans have been cut open, when what's supposed to be inside is suddenly exposed to the outside, and our bio-chemistry and physiology is perturbed. Childbirth and surgery were for centuries feared for their dreadful risks. But worst of all is war. In the First World War, we learned how to save lives by treating injuries at the point of wounding. But losing a limb rather than a life on a battlefield that had once and for a very long time been a manured farm field meant horrendous levels of bacteria blasted deep into already damaged soft tissue and organs. Such exposure was unmanageable, even with the most diligent nursing and the most well-meaning sur-geries, which cut more and more infected flesh away, only for the rot to return. If we want to know what a pre-antibiotic age really looks (and smells) like, then we should go to a field hospital on the Western Front in 1917. The fourth Horseman hangs around, waiting for the lives he should have been able to collect on the battlefield, but he's patient, and he gets many of them eventually anyway, thanks to the second Horseman carrying the pestilence of bacterial infection into what was left of the survivors' bodies.

The sheer volume and horror of infected wound injury in the Great War drove the transformation of antibacterial therapies. On the Allied side, Alexander Fleming worked in a laboratory in the attic of a casino on the French coast, which had been converted into a military hospital. He stayed there for the entire course of the war, looking for an answer, and he spoke about it in his Nobel Prize acceptance lecture: 'Since the war of 1914–18 [I have] been interested in antiseptics.'[83] The war, despite the numbers of casualties, generated no pharmacological breakthrough, but there was a paradigm shift in thinking and research, because of the nature of modern artillery casualty, which involved complex trauma: deep, jagged wounds, twisting through soft tissue into body cavities, and swamped with bacteria and poison. Fleming realized that it was never going to be enough just to treat these injuries topically by sluicing them clean. Bacterial infections would need to be dealt with systemically, from the inside out.[84] At the same time, on the other side of the combatant line, a German biochemist, Gerhard Domagk, learned the same lessons. Domagk was quicker off the mark than Fleming to produce an actual treatment, combining the antiseptic chemicals used to clean wounds from the outside with a synthetic version of the antimalarial quinine, which meant they could be taken safely as medication.[85]

It was Domagk's sulpha drug class that provided the first systemic therapeutic response to bacterial infection. Sulphonamides have been largely forgotten about now, but doctors at the time were astounded at their ability to fight back against diseases like scarlet fever (which kills Beth March in the novel *Little Women*) and puerperal sepsis, both of which were almost always fatal. Obstetricians and gynaecologists had faced nearly as much death and suffering in their civilian wards as the doctors in the field hospitals during the First World War: women dying wretchedly just after giving birth; christenings and funerals on the same day. And sulpha drugs brought almost instant improvements – in 1935, one British obstetrician called it 'the dawn of curative medicine'.[86] Humans were now winning battles in the war they had been losing for their entire existence, no matter whose flag they fought under. But it wasn't quite the new

dawn everyone had hoped for. Sulphonamides were agents of bac-
teriostasis (bacteria inhibiting), not bacteriocide (death to bacteria,
most of them). Patients could be allergic to the sulpha drugs, and
bacteria didn't stay static for very long. Although they worked with
some conditions, it was only a few (and they were mostly suffered
by women and children; no one ever makes medical history just
by doing that). And Domagk made his breakthrough just as Hitler
took power in Germany, and he was working for a pharmaceutical
company, Bayer, which became part of IG Farben, which would go
on to provide much of the industrial infrastructure of Nazism. The
Nazi government forbade him to accept the Nobel Prize he won
for discovering sulpha drugs in 1939, and he was unable to go on to
develop their pharmacological potential (although we still use sulpha
drugs today, in limited settings). So the history of our victory over
bacterial infections became about Fleming discovering penicillin on
his windowsill at St Mary's Hospital in 1928, and then, eventually,
in 1941, a team led by Howard Florey, Ernst Chain and Norman
Heatley was able to concentrate the substance, stabilize it and turn
it into a bacteriocidal drug, and use it on patients, five of whom
indisputably did not die of conditions that previously would have
killed them.[87] It was the dawn of the first age of antibiotics and it
felt almost like something magical was happening.

Here's how antibiotics work: they prevent bacteria from reproducing. Stop something reproducing long enough and it is eventually
destroyed. Antibiotic drugs are designed to undermine the basic

structure and biological processes of the bacteria cell to a point where it is dead. There are three main ways they can do this: they can break down the cell walls that hold all the pieces of the bacterium (a single component of bacteria) together; they can destroy the proteins that do the work of growing the bacteria; or they can work at the genetic level, by targeting the DNA strands with which the bacteria itself is made. All antibiotics do one of these three things, and some of them (the heavy-duty broad-spectrum antibiotics) do all three at the same time. And the principle is sound. If something can't reproduce itself, when it dies, there is nothing left. Not unliving, not held in stasis – dead and gone. With bacterial infection manageable, medicine can get on with whatever else needs to be done to save the human life under threat.

This first age of antibiotics was utterly transforming. It really was the dawn of a new curative age, revolutionizing healthcare and underpinning many of the medical advances of the twentieth century.[88] Childbirth became safe, surgery could become elective, intensive care could truly be intensive. We quickly learned not to fear medical procedures anymore, because whatever their complications might be, antibiotics would save us. We took them for chest infections, which stopped being potentially fatal and became just chest infections. We took them prophylactically to prepare for surgeries, so any bacteria lurking around wouldn't surge into the wound site and take control. We learned to ask for them, and doctors learned to give them to us because it was quick and cheap. If in doubt, take an antibiotic. And we made them an intrinsic part of modern animal husbandry, so pigs, cows and chickens didn't get the kind of infections that animals get and pass around when they are farmed cheaply and intensively in cramped spaces.

The first age was when we also began to discover that there really is no such thing as a completely bacteriocidal antibiotic. However strong the drugs to kill off infections are, however dead the dead ones are, no antibiotic ever quite kills them all. In the first years of the age, this didn't matter, because holding the infection at bay gives the sick human being enough time to develop an immune response of their own to what's left of the infection. But, increasingly, this is no longer the case. Even if only a few bacteria are left behind after a course of antibiotics, under selective pressure the survivors learn to resist, to alter their DNA so they can repair their cell walls and make other proteins so they can reproduce again. The next version of themselves comes with the new learning already incorporated. It's this new version that resurges through the body, resisting whatever is used against it when the symptoms of infection reoccur. We're all familiar with needing one, then a second, then perhaps a third course of a different, increasingly strong antibiotic to cure an infection. That's bacteria learning – and not just from themselves, keeping it in the family. When bacteria die, from whatever cause, they leave a debris of proteins and DNA lying around. Related bacteria types can absorb this – usefully, with the learning intact. Recent research has found that completely unrelated bacteria can also pick up other bacterial family leftovers and absorb them, and absorb all their learning about resistance. Think of it as the microbiological equivalent of downloading a constantly updated new resistance app.[89] All of this is what we now call antibiotic (or antimicrobial) resistance. Penicillin-resistant bacteria strains were detected within a year of penicillin being used, even while everyone thought the magic of antibiotics was strong enough to last forever. But the signs were already there that the first age was always going to be short.

When you've evolved from a planet's earliest prebiotic chemical states, you've had a good long time to learn defensive and resistance mechanisms, and puny human timescales are nothing by comparison.[90] But, for us, the speed at which bacteria adapted to our antibacterial therapies is awesome. The first age of antibiotics lasted about fifty years and was resourced and simultaneously doomed by the pharmaceutical industry's intensive production of the new drug class. Antibiotics produced on an industrial scale generate a like-for-like response from the bacteria they target: antibiotic resistance is also generated on an industrial scale. Scale up one, scale up the other. Speed up usage, speed up resistance. Globalize usage, globalize resistance. Whatever doesn't kill them really does make them stronger. The same goes for antibiotics used on an industrial scale on non-humans in factory farms. We're doing better about not using antibiotics in agriculture, but our primary aim is to make intensive farming more sustainable, not to provide a solution to the problem of resistance. Resistance isn't the fault of farm animals. We did this to ourselves. As one of the leading authorities on infectious diseases says: 'The predominant driver of antibiotic resistance [as it affects] humans is the intense pressure exerted by the misuse and overuse of antibiotics in people.'[91] What all this means is that we, the people, are now living in the second age of antibiotics, where the infections we catch are much smarter than they used to be, and the things we take to cure them work much less well, and there's no more magic.

The second age of antibiotics means we are learning to fear bacteria again. Sound the alarm, as the rider of the white horse gallops into view! He's finding more and more space to roam across the second age of antibiotics, and a whole new class of weapons to use against us, most of which we've handed to him ourselves. None of these weapons is more powerful than *Acinetobacter baumannii*.*[92] *Acinetobacter baumannii* is one of the most troublesome pathogens for healthcare institutions and their patients, wherever they are in the world.[93] There are times when scientific language is both precise and dramatic at the same time. One of those is when microbiologists write in otherwise impenetrably complicated clinical microbiology journals about *Acinetobacter baumannii*. They've called the observation of its level of resistance to antibiotics 'a sentinel event'. 'Sentinel' is a word with general and medical meanings. In general terms, a sentinel stands watch for danger, guarding a border behind which those they protect are gathered. Medically, a sentinel event means imminent danger of disease or a condition that possibly means death.[94] Whatever meaning you choose, sentinel events mean pay attention – PAY ATTENTION. Imminent threat, imminent threat of death – even if other imminent threats seem to

---

* Pronounced 'bow-man-ee-eye', and named for the microbiologist, Paul Baumann, who identified it as a separate type in 1968.

be more imminent, they are nothing compared to the strength and the patience of *Acinetobacter baumanii.*

Acinetobacter baumannii is an opportunistic pathogen – which means it can only be contracted by people who are already ill, wounded or physiologically 'perturbed', so already on antibiotics, or immune compromised.[95] It isn't yet hanging around on street corners, waiting to pounce on the healthy. It is a biofilm bacterial form.[96] Researchers who work on nothing else used to say that it was resistant to a wide range of antibiotics. Now they say that it is resistant to all known antibiotics. Nothing can stop it. There's almost admiration in their tone when they describe how quickly *Acinetobacter baumannii* adapts to everything humans can throw at it, how impressive it is at finding new ways to respond swiftly to changes in selective environmental pressure. How, like all biofilms, it has evolved to use its rate of gene exchange – swapping out non-useful genes for useful ones – faster and more effectively than its fellows, and how it's one of those bacteria that can use genes from outside the *Acinetobacter* family to grow stronger. And each survey, each genome sequence, each molecular epidemiological technique applied to understanding its mechanisms concludes the same thing: that *Acinetobacter baumannii* has outstanding potential to survive and grow more resistant, whereas we, as yet, have little to offer in our own defence. Scientists talk about its 'uncanny ability' to survive for prolonged periods, in hostile environments.[97] Uncanny abilities are those that mystify scientists, mostly because they don't understand what it is to survive for two billion years in hot pools of varying salinity on our planet.

What they know for our time is that *Acinetobacter baumannii* loves a hospital-bed handrail, especially if it's in a burns ward or a critical care ward, full of really sick patients with open wounds and constant dressing changes, or a place with humans on ventilators, and no matter how hard those wards are cleaned, how closely the cracks and crevices and corners are scrubbed, *Acinetobacter baumannii* hangs on. It's been found on humidifiers, urine-collection jugs and computer keyboards, all of which had been previously and scrupulously cleaned. There is a machine called a pulsatile lavage kit that fires antiseptic liquid at an open wound site under pressure, like putting your thumb over a hose so the water comes out more strongly, and sluices out hard-to-reach debris. Pulsatile lavage kits are an efficient way to manage wounds that need constant care before surgical repair, except that the equipment itself poses a significant risk of transmission of resistant *Acinetobacter baumannii*, squirting it deep into a wound that's about to be made bigger, deliberately.[98] Once *Acinetobacter baumannii* is in, then it sweeps round the body, infecting the blood, the brain, the lungs and (favourite of so many bacteria strains) the urinary tract. And on it goes. *Acinetobacter baumannii* survives being dried out (desiccated) better than other types of bacteria. It can survive being airborne – so it may not be motile, but it travels. It's now thought that 80 per cent of all *Acinetobacter* infections are *Acinetobacter baumannii*. It's almost as if all the other fifteen different types of *Acinetobacter* have given up.[99]

Perhaps the most uncanny thing about it is that, for most of humanity's time on the planet, *Acinetobacter baumannii* has been a benign soil dweller.[100] It lived, without really bothering us, on the land we farmed and made our livings from, a non-opportunistic biofilm made of colonies of round individual bacteria. It's probably something to do with temperature and nutrition. Soil is cooler than humans; things that live in it don't need to eat so much to live. Fewer messages skip between the exterior and interior cells. Live and let live. Somewhere on the planet, the benign soil dweller found its way into a human, and it was first registered in American hospitals in the late 1980s. There was no particular concern about the presence of this strain of bacteria in the medical space, because new antibiotics could always be discovered to deal with it, or existing ones tweaked, and it mostly infected patients whose outlook was pretty grim anyway.

Then, in 2003, as the rider of the blood-red horse is happy to remind us, the US and its allies went to war in Iraq for the second time. *Acinetobacter baumannii* lived in the sand and soil in Iraq, as it always had done, benignly, resisting what it needed to, which wasn't very much, officially designated non-virulent. And trampling over the ground came soldiers, and after them came explosive weapons. These were different from the mechanisms of injury that had been seen in the first Iraq war, in 1990, and they were much more like those of the First World War. The artillery and improvised explosive devices (IEDs) blew huge holes in human soft tissue, wounding down to their body cavities, blasting soil debris containing *Acinetobacter baumannii* deep inside their bodies. Casualties had very brief stays in a field hospital, long enough for some damage-control surgery and lab work to be done, to see what infections they might be carrying. Then they were loaded into specialist medical-transport aircraft, and their bloodwork results were sent ahead of them, digitally. When they got home for definitive repair, there it was in the pathology report: *Acinetobacter baumannii*.

But in a new biofilm form. The cell walls of the form that lives in soil are translucently thin, because it doesn't need them to be any other way. The form that lives in humans is different. Its cell-capsule walls are thicker, more opaque, stronger. Somehow, in the transfer of the bacteria into humans, a genetic switch had happened, and the biofilm had toughened up, becoming denser, hungrier, resistant to changing temperatures and disinfectants and human immune responses. From there, it wasn't a huge shift for it to become resistant to human antibiotics. By the time the wounded soldiers were taken into critical care wards, along with their infections, *Acinetobacter baumannii* had settled into its new home. Microbiologists began to call it *Iraqibacter*, because it was so prevalent in US and UK returning casualties – or *Ukrainibacter*, for the soldiers wounded and infected in the war in eastern Ukraine in 2014.[101]

Whether military casualties brought *Acinetobacter baumanii* back with them from the war, or whether they caught it from a hospital bed handrail, or a ventilator tube, or a burn dressing, the only solution was to isolate them in single sterile rooms, every surface cleaned within an inch of its – and their – life ('enhanced environmental cleaning to eliminate the organism from the peri-patient environment').[102] Then they were intensively nursed by people wearing something very similar to the armour worn by medics treating Ebola patients – layers of anonymizing plastic between them and another human. Combatting *Acinetobacter baumannii* meant longer stays in hospital than expected, failed operations, massive doses of one kind of antibiotic after another, round and round, until something worked, endlessly testing – and it meant pain, fever, misery. It wasn't just the medical effort they had to endure. Contact isolation is hard – we really understand that now. Just as with viruses, the consequences of infection by a resistant strain of bacteria affect the mental health of sufferers as well as their physical recovery. Isolation is worst of all for those who have already endured war and occupation, because being alone means they think of little else but horrors past, and this is true if the human infected by *Acinetobacter baumannii* is a solder in the military ward in Birmingham, a Syrian citizen made deaf from the constant pounding explosions around them, or a child of Mosul, injured in the aftermath of liberation. If they are lucky, one of the new breed of clinical psychologists will come to their room and explain about antibacterial resistance, adapting their language to the age, educational circumstance and auditory capacity of whoever is in the isolation bed. It's especially hard with children, who need to be encouraged to stay where they are, on their own, and not to run away to try to find their families, and to eat and drink properly, and to please believe that, if they do this, they will get better and will be able to go home.[103]

But home is where people are misusing and overusing antibiotics without any medical supervision, making the crisis of antibacterial resistance worse all on their own, out of their ordinary bathroom cabinets. Urinary tract infections, for instance, are usually caused by *Escherichia coli* (more commonly known as *E. coli*), and it shares many of the features that make *Acinetobacter Baumannii* so feared. Urinary tract infections caused by *E. coli* are the second most common infectious presentation in global community healthcare practice (the most common are upper respiratory tract infections, or, as they are more commonly known, the secondary symptoms of a cold). But many patients don't get as far as their local healthcare centre, because there are medications aimed at treating urinary tract infections that don't need a prescription, or can be bought online.[104] The small print on their packaging tends to say things like, 'helps inhibit the progress of infection', or, 'not intended to replace medical care', or, 'this medicine can't treat an active infection, only control it'. In other, larger words (which aren't on the packet), these drugs are bacteriostatics, so the bacterial infection is not being destroyed, only held at a stop sign. While it waits, selective pressure operates and the bacteria has time to learn how to survive virulently. *E. coli* learns especially fast, so when it's allowed to move once more, and spread back, the consequence is multi-resistant, morbid urinary tract infections that never shift.

The provider of last resort for the elimination of urinary tract infections, once the pharmaceutical options are exhausted, is a urology surgeon. In procedures conducted under general anaesthesia, they scrape clean a urinary tract or a bladder wall as best they know how, hoping that their operating theatre, gown and mask are effective in preventing other bacteria getting through. And then the patient endures a long stay in hospital, most likely in isolation, with no guarantee of a full recovery.[105] All over the hospital, there are fewer guarantees of any kind. Doctors are having to get used to conversations with patients who have survived heart surgery or multiple brutal cycles of chemotherapy and have been declared as recovering, in which they have to tell them that they spoke too soon, that at some point in their treatment or in its aftermath they contracted an infection that simply can't be treated, because they've run out of antibiotic options. And, increasingly, this infection won't just ruin their lives, it will kill them. This is life in the second age.

The second age means that, across the entire world, home- and hospital-grown bacterial resistance increases at scale and pace. We also know that it has country-specific features. Within Switzerland, for instance, antibiotic prescription, usage and misuse varies by canton and language spoken.[106] No one has quite worked out why. In Syria, we have a much better understanding of the reasons for nationally specific bacterial resistance, and it's not for the immediately obvious reason of the now-constant presence of the rider on the blood-red horse. Before he settled in, Syria was a middle-income country, with a functioning healthcare system providing free-at-the-point-of-delivery healthcare services, and a population with a preference for home births.[107] And it saw the same antibiotic complacency and developing antibiotic resistance as every other country in the world, for all the same reasons: excessive, unmonitored antibiotic prescribing, antibiotics available without prescription, and patient over-expectations. Then there were the Syria-specific reasons for the growth of antibiotic resistance. Since the 1980s, the country had developed a significant pharmaceutical industry, with sixty-three factories (subsidized by the Syrian government, many located in and around Aleppo). They produced 5,700 different products, many of them antibiotics. Syria could not only meet its own pharmaceutical needs, it exported to fifty-two other countries, including most of the Middle East.[108] Because so many of them worked in the industry, the Syrian population knew their antibiotics. So they asked their doctors not just for antibiotics, but for specific kinds of antibiotics, by all their complicated antibiotic names: Augmentin (also called co-amoxiclav), meropenem, vancomycin, Tazocin – all broad-spectrum antibiotics, not to be used until all the others have failed. A pre-2011 study of 430 Syrian households showed that 85 per cent of them had used antibiotics in the preceding month, with only 43 per cent of these courses being prescribed by a medical professional.

It was the same story in Syria's hospitals. *Acinetobacter baumannii* was the most common cause of ventilator-based pneumonia across intensive-care units in general hospitals in Damascus. But not just *Acinetobacter baumannii*. There was very little surveillance of hospital-borne infections, and low priority on infection prevention and control. Syria had very few microbiologists, infectious diseases specialists or labs where they could work, because these weren't considered to be speciality areas of training and there was no money in it. Labs were being built, but they were increasingly 'public–private partnerships', with the emphasis on the unregulated private, just like the rest of the healthcare system. Politics made everything in the public health space worse. There was a cholera outbreak in 2008 because the newly privatized water providers weren't doing their job of purification properly, so there was a new layer of gastric infections to cope with, particularly in children, linking up with falling vaccination rates. Syria's citizens were under increasing political and environmental pressure. Few things flourished, apart from the political elite and resistant bacteria strains. Entire bacterial families, including those that cause tonsillitis in children and pneumonia, were becoming almost entirely resistant to antibiotics, including to what are known as the salvage therapy antibiotics – the very broad-spectrum medications that are used on very resistant bacteria as a very last resort.

And then, in 2011, came civil war. The blood-red horse cleared any remaining obstacles in the way of Pestilence and his weapons of resistant bacterial strains. National healthcare collapsed completely.[109] Cities were smashed, but still remained full of people who had nowhere else to go, being joined by thousands of the distressed displaced. Hospitals became field hospitals (and became targets for bombing, whatever side they were on). The safest place to go was underground, but it was only one kind of safe. While the guns and shells pounded overhead, infection was spreading beneath their feet, and up the walls, and everywhere around them. Underground hospitals are difficult to manage bacteriologically. Patients bring in bugs, bugs take up residence, thrive. It happens in well-resourced hospitals above ground, in peace and daylight, no matter how hard we work to keep them out. Imagine if the entry to the medical facility looked like a First World War trench.

In Syria, in the civil war, chemicals like chlorine that were needed to sterilize medical instruments and hospital wards were hard to come by, and some of the time they were not available at all – often being confiscated in case the plan was to use them to make chemical weapons, rather than to clean surgical instruments or for wiping down hospital bed handrails. Even if the chemicals were available, increasing interruption of electrical power meant machines couldn't run, water was cold and lighting was done by generators, flickering and dim. And, in the meantime, patients kept coming. Water plants were bombed, so waterborne infections spread, all of them in forms resistant to most antibiotics, and every day another drug got added to the 'tried it, it failed' list. We monitor attacks on hospitals as best we can, and we should add attacks on utilities as well, as part of the broader healthcare infrastructure. No water, no power, more bacterial infections, more resistant, untreatable strains.

And wounds – the constant of all kinds of war, no matter where or when. Almost every kind of weapon has been used in the course of the Syrian civil war, from high-velocity sniper rifle fire targeting heads and spines, to huge bombs in heavy air-strikes that destroyed buildings and the people in them, blasting them open, smashing them with fragments and burning their skin and their lungs. Wounded patients presented to whatever kind of facility could call itself a hospital, straight from the attack or months afterwards. Most difficult to deal with were those who had external bone fixators holding together broken limbs, where rusty, hastily inserted metal parts had taken infections right to the bone, in a straight line, no dawdling around in soft tissue along the way. Prescriptions and treatments with antibiotics became guesswork, using what was left in the stores and knowing that none of the kit in the hospital, from catheters to ventilators, was clean enough to be inserted into a human being. And what was left in the stores might be more trouble than it was worth. Stocks from the sixty-three pharmaceutical factories, including billions of tablets in blister packs, were swilling around in the chaos, just waiting to be stolen, bartered, smuggled. Their boxes were copied and stuffed with fakes, sold on the black market. Fake or genuine, if they were all that was to hand, people took them, sold them, prescribed them, no matter what, because it felt like they were at least doing something – antibiotics taken in lieu of a healthcare system (more about that later) – and all the old habits of mis- or overuse of the medications were made harder by war.

One of the few medical networks left functional in Syria by 2017 was that of the pharmacies, and when they keep going, there is always hope. Pharmacists had become the first and only point of contact for most of the sick, giving out advice and selling medications, including antibiotics. Three newly graduated Syrian pharmacists were talking, and they came to realize two things. Firstly, the civil war had significantly increased their country's problem with antimicrobial resistance. And secondly, during the whole of their medical education, Syrian pharmacists received no teaching or information whatsoever about antimicrobial resistance. So the three of them approached the Syrian Pharmacists Association, which still had a scientific committee, and asked if they could try to fix at least part of the problem. If pharmacists could understand antimicrobial resistance, then they could make sure they were selling the right drug for the actual condition presented to them by their customer-patients. The campaign was approved, and the three pharmacists became nineteen volunteers, who went out to spread the message not just to pharmacies, but to healthcare centres and some hospitals in Damascus.

They set off to travel around a city whose outer suburbs were part of the civil war, and where ISIS and al-Qaeda regularly set off bombs. Even on less explosive days, there was still danger, with the constant threat of arrest and detention, absolute uncertainty and very high strain. Nevertheless, they found their way to 413 pharmacies (half of all pharmacies in the entire city) and spoke to them. They gave them materials, fliers, links to a Facebook page, and small, specially printed cards that they in turn could give out to their patient-customers, explaining why they had been given antibiotics and how important it was to use them properly, to finish the course, and not to let anyone else take the medication.[110] Beyond Syria, we've begun to develop the concept of 'the persuasive pharmacy'. Pharmacists speak to patients to try to work out exactly what their symptoms are, and what medications it would be best for them to take in order to get better. If a patient has the proper prescription for antibiotics, the pharmacist will remind them how to take them, that they should finish the course and not stop once they feel better, and that they certainly shouldn't keep some for when they have something like a tickly throat in the future. Persuasive pharmacists are well represented by the nineteen volunteers in Damascus. Pharmacists generally have a lot of patience and excellent communication skills, and they are committed and courageous. It would be good if there were some equivalent persuasive-pharmacy chatbot that chimed in every time someone went to buy antibiotics on the Internet.

There is a technical term for this kind of activity, wherever it is done: antibiotic stewardship. Like 'sentinels', 'stewardship' has both a general meaning and a specific medical interpretation. Here is its official definition: 'Antimicrobial stewardship is a coherent set of actions that promote using antimicrobials responsibly.'*[111]

My colleague, Dr Esmita Charani, is the steward I know best. Esmita trained as a pharmacist, and spent the first ten years of her career working in hospitals, watching the first age of antibiotics turn into the second age. She went back to university to get post-graduate degrees in infectious diseases and medical anthropology. Let's unpick her decision carefully. Firstly, infectious diseases: this is an obvious choice for a pharmacist with an interest in bacterial pathogens. When she began her infectious diseases research work, she was part of a team that wrote one of the very first academic papers to analyse 'the development and implementation of a smartphone application for the delivery of antimicrobial prescribing policy'.[112] She still works on today's apps, and the issues of governance and oversight that will be needed for the apps of the future. She contributes to precise analysis and guidance on improving prescription practices, to encourage prudent use of antibiotics. She's studying and testing the redesigning of what she calls 'the choice architecture of hospital prescription charts' – discussing what the ideal chart would look like, that doesn't push a busy doctor to imprudent antibiotic use. She has worked on analysis that establishes the frameworks for better, shorter use of specific antibiotics. She's researched how some instruments are easier to keep sterile than others. While I

---

* It only has this interpretation in relation to antimicrobial resistance. We don't need to secure stewardship of other kinds of drugs because they don't pose a risk to both the treated individual *and* the community, so we don't have antihistamine stewardship, for instance.

have known her, she has done all of this in laboratories at St Mary's Hospital in London, a few hundred yards from Alexander Fleming's original peacetime workplace.

Then there is her less conventional decision to study medical anthropology (although the interest in designing the choice architecture of prescription charts is a bit of a giveaway). Medical anthropology looks at the many different ways that decisions are made about health and treatment, and it has a particular interest in the language used around medicine. In addition to the science of bacterial infection, what Esmita has become most interested in – and alarmed by – is how human communication, face to face, is such a significant factor in the strengthening of antibiotic resistance. The issue is not doctor/pharmacist-to-patient communication, but communication among doctors themselves, especially in hospitals with very ill human beings who are likely to end up in those post-operative or critical care wards where the challenge of antimicrobial resistance is strongest.

In 2019, Esmita and colleagues completed an ethnographical study of antibiotic decision-making in a big London hospital (sometimes fieldwork is done by going down a couple of floors in the main lift). They identified twenty-three key medical staff to follow around, some who did acute surgery and some acute medical work. With the right consents, they watched patients all the way along their pathway through the hospital, from emergency admittance to general ward and discharge. They scrubbed up and went into operating theatres. They joined in ward rounds. They observed multidisciplinary team meetings, where patient progress and likely outcomes were discussed. They followed trolleys as patients were moved from ward to ward, and they watched the medical handovers – when records, lists and updates were passed from night teams to day teams, surgery teams to ward teams, in corridors, meeting rooms or outside lifts. They were careful to blend in, so that, as far as possible, their twenty-three subjects forgot they were there, until they asked them to explain the medical decisions they had just made.[113]

Esmita was lead author on the report where the findings were published in 2019, and those findings were clear. The first twenty-four hours of admission are the most important of all if infection is to be diagnosed and managed successfully. But there are multiple teams involved in this period and it is very difficult to sustain prescription control. Emergency department antibiotic prescription is often good, if on the strong side (usually due to worries about sepsis – rightly so, because this inflammatory response to blood-borne infection is a quick killer). When the patient is then moved to surgery or a ward, this would be a good place to ask if they need to continue on strong, clobber-everything antibiotics, or if treatment can be de-escalated. De-escalation is always a good thing in antibiotic stewardship. Less is more (putting it medically, shorter courses of targeted antibiotics work better than long courses of broad-spectrum ones).[114] But often this doesn't happen. Antibiotic treatment keeps getting moved to the back of the queue for attention, and usually ends up being done last of all, by junior staff, who prescribe defensively (too many antibiotics, broad-spectrum, and usually for too long). This is wrong, and increasingly dangerous. In the second age of antibiotics, staying on the safe side isn't really safe anymore.

Esmita's study was the first, but their findings from one London hospital about the dangers of late, defensive antibiotic prescribing are now 'emerging themes' (which means people are paying attention), and the same results come from all the replica studies, from India to Australia. There are some practical steps that can be implemented quickly: a checklist, specifically about antibiotic prescribing, that is begun in the admitting department and remains with the patient for the length of their stay. Ideally, the checklist is overseen by someone on the medical team whose primary, dedicated role is to have continuous antimicrobial oversight of the patient, all the way along their treatment pathway. They hold a checklist and a digital dashboard, so they can see at a glance how many patients are being administered which antibiotics in their hospital and if they need to do anything about any of them. To put it untechnically, a steward doing stewardship.

Checklists, dashboards and dedicated roles all work well in theory, and hopefully in practice. What mostly stops them working well is the level of communication they require across professional and institutional boundaries. Someone is always the most senior person in the room, and they may have other priorities than antimicrobial stewardship. Telling them which prescription to write for antibiotics, or to work with the much more junior doctor who will be writing one, or telling them they are writing the wrong one, an old-fashioned one that doesn't work anymore – all of these things can be hard and feel like professional transgression. Medical disciplines have their own cultures of authority, their own languages. Whoever the steward is, they'll need to learn all of them, and be able to be firm but authoritative, because they are holding the line, and it breaks if they do, first and worst of all in hospitals. Somewhere at the heart of stewardship should always be the ability to speak truth to power when it comes to antibiotic resistance, and it encourages others to develop the courage to save by speaking out. Stewardship is saying very loudly and clearly that it is dangerous if antibiotic decision-making is somehow seen as less important than surgery. Stewardship sounds the sentinel warning that eventually this leads to doctors having to explain to patients that, yes, their surgery was successful, but, no, they are not getting any better, because their post-operatively acquired infection can no longer be managed with antibiotics, because bacteria in and beyond the hospital have learned resistance in the meantime.

During the COVID pandemic, Esmita set aside much of her research and went back into the part of the hospital where she had begun her medical career. Pharmacists looked for new lines they could hold in places that they already knew, like the hospital dispensary, where they created and maintained aseptic areas so they could make up intravenous medications that were ready for immediate use by individual patients, so nursing staff didn't have to spend more time off ward than necessary. They prepared ready-to-use injectables for the same reason (and both these developments are likely to become the standard in the NHS, post-pandemic). They developed new pharmacy storage areas as wards moved around and the medication offering for COVID patients grew and moved with them. As they went along, they learned about the critical care of patients, and many of them did some basic critical care ward training to enhance their support of their nursing colleagues. As COVID wards (always critical care wards) grew or needed to be moved to other parts of the hospital, pharmacists could help with the physical process of making routes between floors and wards clean and safe and clutter free, becoming part of the team that physically moved each patient.[115] Pharmacists, no one should be surprised to learn, were flexible and committed and imaginative and collaborative in finding solutions and closing gaps. When this is over, we'll all benefit from the new lines they laid down that make hospital critical care pathways run more smoothly. And all while keeping vigilant against the possibility of secondary bacterial infection that might require antibiotics and produce a surge of its own in antimicrobial resistance, remaining part of the global community of stewards, holding that section of the line.

There is a fine line between good stewardship communication prac- tices and lecturing people who have very few other choices about proper and responsible antibiotic use. It runs through places, like civil-war-wrecked Syria, where antibiotics are taken in lieu of what is left of their healthcare system. Even in countries with no ability to manufacture their own pharmaceuticals, antibiotics are seldom in short supply, even when everything else is.[116] Boxes of all kinds pile up in medical-facility stockrooms and pharmacies – quick, cheap and easy to supply by aid agencies, NGOs, private companies and donors, who still work from the ideal and the simplicity of the first age of antibiotics. It's common for doctors in very under-resourced medical units, when they hear something through their stethoscope that might be a respiratory infection in the lungs of a child, to prescribe an antibiotic without ever identifying what bacteria are actually causing the problem. Sometimes, they prescribe several antibiotics at the same time, because they have them and they can, and because it's doing something, when the alternative is nothing. In adults, urinary tract infections are confused with STIs, but the response is the same: an antibiotic, and then another one the next day, until the patient's symptoms seem to be clearing up. Esmita is very clear about how we need to understand this process, and about how there are many different dynamics by which stewardship is achieved. For patients and doctors in these countries, 'antibiotics are progress . . . antibiotics represent inclusion in modernity'. As long as the doctor can give them the box of tablets, the healthcare system is functioning. And, some of the time, they work. The patient can go home, until their next cough or pain gets serious enough to seek medical help again, and in the meantime, resistance grows, so the next dosage of pills may not work as well, and then, one day, not at all. All over the world, antimicrobial resistance is like a song with multiple different verses in many different languages, but all with the same chorus: in the meantime, resistance grows, and one day our means to combat bacterial infection may no longer work at all.

If using antibiotics in lieu of a healthcare system was something that happened accidentally, it's becoming more formalized now. There have been several scientific studies that have looked at what happens if antibiotics are given prophylactically – to prevent disease before it even happens. Some of the results look like magic. Azith-romycin is an antibiotic that is used to treat a range of bacterial infections, including those of the middle ear, gastrointestinal infec-tions, pneumonia and those related to malaria. A research study was instigated where it was given to children prophylactically – before they had reported symptoms of anything – across sub-Saharan Africa, and mortality fell by as much as 22 per cent. Another antibiotic, amoxicillin, was given to mothers in the UK about to give birth with surgical assistance, to prevent post-delivery infections (that Fleming and Domagk would have recognized as puerperal fever). More magic. Infection rates fell, and the authors of the study immediately recommended that the WHO should change its guidance so that giving prophylactic antibiotics to women likely to undergo surgical intervention in childbirth should be routine.

But, across the world, the scientific and stewardship jury is very much out on what the results actually mean. Neither trial looked at whether strengthening public-health measures to control possible infections – such as hygiene, clean water, antisepsis practice and (in the case of the African study) mosquito nets to prevent malaria – would have been equally effective. Neither trial lasted long enough to look at the possible effects of prophylaxis on resistance. In sub-Saharan Africa, this was especially relevant, because azithromycin is used extensively and effectively against trachoma, a particularly nasty form of infectious blindness that causes scarring of the eyelid. Treatment and sanitation improvements have almost obliterated the bacteria from the region – a great example of how antibiotics, used with care and in conjunction with public-health measures, can be transforming – but the trial might increase resistant forms of the bacteria, and then new forms of trachoma would come back and all the work would be undone. And other stewards, looking at the study in India, worried about the effects of perinatal antibiotics on the health of babies, and the possible negative implications for the intergenerational transfer of beneficial human microbes. They have strongly urged the WHO to hold off on any change in their recommendations. What these studies mean is that we are still hoping the magic of the first age of the antibiotic can be recreated in places where the healthcare system is mostly absent. That's the dilemma of antibiotics being present. It's a space where stewardship is essential and stewards are the best people to do the hard thinking, and to help the rest of us to understand.[117]

If we are currently living in the second age of antibiotics, what does this mean the third age will be? The third age of antibiotics is the one where they don't work anymore. Where they become sidelined, a mostly redundant mechanism to mitigate bacterial infection. The third age is when we find out what we are going to use instead of antibiotics, when we see what science may have in store for us. There are several research tracks underway that have the potential to find an alternative to antibiotics, so let's follow them as far as they go today.

Firstly, phage therapy. Bacteriophage translates as 'bacteria-eater', and the entity doing the eating is a virus that attacks bacteria from within. We haven't yet worked out if they are actually life forms, so if they actually eat things, or in some other unlife-form way consume them. A very few of us have known about them since the early twentieth century, when scientists identified particular entities, which they called bacteriophages, that appeared to be living parasites of bacteria, although they didn't do much with the information, because many of the concepts of the microbiological world were so new to us. We've gone back to looking at the possibility of phage therapy in particular because of cystic fibrosis (CF), where a genetic condition causes the sufferer's lungs to constantly fill up with thick, easily infected mucus. The worst infection is caused by the bacterium *Pseudomonas aeruginosa*, which is opportunistic, very resistant and (unsurprisingly) a biofilm. It's dangerous to anyone in critical care and almost half of all cystic fibrosis sufferers get it. Because it is so quick to adapt to new living conditions, residual infections of *Pseudomonas aeruginosa* can hang on even after double lung transplants have, in all other ways, transformed the lives of CF patients. Phages work against bacteria because they seem to be able to get through bacterial biofilm walls, and then to stimulate what are called the suicide or death genes of bacteria – so, when they die, they really die. (No one is really sure why bacteria have death genes; it might be something to do with the way they communicate in biofilms to maintain their overall group health.[118]) We also don't know how phages are going to work on humans overall, because they currently consist of quite strongly toxic compounds. We don't know if their effects can be sustained, or if bacteria develop phage resistance. We don't know how to administer a drug we haven't finished inventing yet, and it will almost certainly require nanotechnology, which is never a quick thing to realize.[119]

Then there is the antibacterial research activity that seeks to enhance processes already at work in our bodies. These include antibody treatments, which we all understand a little better in 2021. Antibodies are part of our own immune response: a protein found in blood, which defends us from foreign bodies, like viruses and bacteria. Antibodies seek them out and wrap around them, stopping them from reproducing or getting a hold on potential hosts. Llamas have a special kind of antibody in their llama blood which helps them resist infection by coating, for instance, spiky virus shapes so they are unable to latch on to their body's organs. Like the bats with the self-modulating immune systems, this may have to do with llamas evolving to live efficiently at altitude in the Andes, and we might one day be able to adapt the model for human use (zoonosis goes both ways).[120] Humans already use antibody therapies effectively in treatments for cancer and other complex conditions, but we have much further to go if we want to use them against resistant strains of bacteria. There are a number of antibody-based antibacterials currently in testing, and what we know so far is that they seem to be working, but only against the specific single bacteria type for which they have been designed.[121] Any antibody-based antibacterial will need to be given early in the infection, so not only do we need to know exactly what strain of bacteria it is, we also need to have the antibody therapy ready to go, straight away, properly targeted. This kind of ultra-fast precision medicine is very challenging, and also not a quick thing to realize.

Harnessing our own microbiological capabilities is also being worked on by scientists exploring the potential of our microbiome.

The microbiome is the genetic underlay of all the microbes that make up our body – bacteria, fungi (more about that in the Famine section), viruses and yeasts. There are layers of microbiome everywhere within us, but particularly in our stomachs, and it's very particular to us, which means that it could be used to design completely individual therapies against things like resistant bacteria strains, especially those which target us through our gastrointestinal system. To do this, we would have to be able to map our individual microbiomes, fill in any gaps and vulnerabilities that resistant bacteria could exploit, and thereby strengthen our own defence mechanism. We are in the early stages of being able to transplant microbiomes from one human to another, but so far that hasn't worked ideally.[122] It all sounds promising, but we'll need huge, very expensive instruments to map the microbiome, and, although one day they may be smaller and cheaper and transportable to any medical facility in the world, that day, too, is a long way off. And we can't yet read the entire microbiome – even microbiome scientists have compared this space in humans to 'dark matter', which isn't great branding. We know dark matter is present in the universe because it exerts gravitational influence on galaxies. We've got some sense of why and what it does, but we can't see it, and it's been really hard to image it.[123] It's much the same with our microbiomes; mostly what we know is that there are 'multiple levels of the unknown'.[124]

And what all of these theoretical therapies that might mean the dawn of the third age have in common is that, even in their most well-conceived form, they are still adjuvants. 'Adjuvant' sounds like 'adjunct', and that's more or less what they are. In medicine, adjuvants are used alongside other drugs to help them do the heavy lifting against diseases and infections. Any therapy that is an adjuvant therapy against bacterial infection still needs an antibiotic to do the hard work. These are all exciting fields of research, and we need to keep doing them, even if it's expensive and difficult and time-consuming. We also need to remember that, at this stage, it's all science and not yet medicine. Medical research in its earliest forms is generally referred to as being preclinical. Research into non-antibiotic-based infection therapeutics is pre-preclinical. And when it comes to thinking about preclinical applications, just working out how each one should be tested will be extremely challenging. So, whichever way we come at it, what all of this means is that the second age of antibiotics will need to be a very long one, just to find out if a third age is even going to be possible.

So, that's what we should be aiming for: to make the second age last as long as possible. Within the antibiotic paradigm, much of the research is devoted to combating the biofilm to end all bio-films, *Acinetobacter baumannii*. When the microbiologists identified the means whereby *Acinetobacter baumannii* switches on its virulence to move from soil to human pestilence, they also identified the potential to switch it off. Those bacteria that threaten us most of all are dependent on the biofilm lifestyle. Breaking up biofilms so they aren't a functioning matrix or colony would have 'immense implications for the treatment of microbial infections'.[125] If we can do it to *Acinetobacter baumannii*, we can do it to any of them. Sentinels can work both ways. We've identified the language biofilm bacteria use to communicate and develop. Perhaps one day we'll learn to speak it enough to tell them to flick off their switches, interrupt their communication, stay where they are, as they are.

And, while we fish about in biofilm bacterial DNA to look for virulence switches, we can make their lives much less comfortable than they are now. While we work to strengthen places like our microbiome so we become a less comfortable environment for bacteria to flourish in, we also want to transform the inanimate environment, where bacterial biofilms live and wait on everything from indwelling medical prostheses to bedrails to flexible plastic hospital water pipes. Especially water pipes. The point at which water is pumped into hospitals is always precarious; this is obviously the case when it's been bombed into dysfunction, or the water purifi-cation system behind it has been destroyed, but it's also a problem in normal, everyday, well-resourced hospitals. The flexible ridged pipes that go round corners inside the foundations of buildings are easy and quick and cheap to install, and they never wear out, but they allow bacterial growth to flourish in all those ridges, and they are difficult to keep really clean. Resistant bacterial biofilms, from the outside and the inside, find an affordable home in the plastic piping of every hospital, and waterborne resistant bacteria can drip from every tap, getting left behind as droplets dry out.

So, apart from ever more zealous and heavy cleaning regimes, part of our response is to create antimicrobial surfaces on the things we use in hospitals. We have known about materials that bacteria don't like for almost as long as we have known about bacteria. We use silver across our medical systems because it inhibits bacterial growth and promotes healing. Fine coatings of silver are applied on invasive medical technology, and we can buy silver-coated sticking plasters for our own wounds in pharmacies. Copper is particularly dangerous for biofilms. Its surface degrades bacterial membranes and damages their DNA. The UK government recommendation for hospitals putting in new water pipes is *not* to use flexible, ridged, bendy plastic piping, but to use either straight plastic, even though it makes construction difficult, or copper, even though it is expensive. Neither copper nor silver is cheap, even in alloys, and both are a finite resource on our planet, the mining of which is environmentally damaging. It's also quite hard, and weird, to imagine what a mostly copper hospital ward would look like.

It's not so much other material alternatives to copper and silver that we're looking for, it's models for the surface that are hostile to bacteria, especially in biofilm formation. We've found them in natural smart surfaces that we already know are antimicrobial. Cicada wings, for instance. Cicadas are fascinating from whichever angle you study them (their life cycles are unorthodox and they make the loud clicking and buzzing noises that soundtrack much of the night-time in warmer parts of the world). But their wings are best of all. Cicada wings are transparent, clear membranes, supported by fine black edging, like tiny stained-glass windows. The material is very fine, and the slightest dirty bacterial fleck sticking to it would disrupt their flight. So, cicada wings are covered in spikes, and the spikes are so small – nanoscale small – they puncture bacterial cell walls and kill them, and the bacteria falls away. Cicada wings are very sterile places. Something similar happens with sharks; although we like to imagine their skin is kept clean by all those little fish nibbling away at the dead bits, it's actually the very special kind of surface roughness of their skin that keeps it really clean. It's a topography that bacteria find very stressful to settle on; it's uncomfortable, distracting, and means they can't get on and build a biofilm. So, rather than persist, the bacteria go looking for somewhere else to live. We can model what these antimicrobial surfaces look like, and then we can manufacture them and stick them to things, making self-cleaning, anti-adhesive places where bacteria would rather not be. There's much less of a welcome for *Acinetobacter baumannii* on a smart-surfaced hospital-ward handrail.

There are other ways to make smart surfaces self-cleaning, using chemicals that are triggered by light, but we aren't quite sure what the long-term effects of their usage might be. Nature has helpfully been testing the antibacterial properties of cicada wings and shark skin for eons, so we know they work safely. And we can 3D print functional nanomaterial composites (a solid material made up of multiple dimensions of useful things, all less than a hundred nanometres wide) in other parts of the university to produce useful smart sheets that can be cut to size and shape. Eventually those could be applied to surfaces that need to be smarter about bacteria living on them. But we can't do both of those things in the same place, yet. And the timescales for us being able to do that are, well, preclinical. Everyone involved in the smart-surfaces field wants us not to be distracted by the images of shark skin and cicada wing, and to remember the timescales. The long second age will eventually incorporate smart antibacterial surfaces, and they will be cheap to produce and readily adaptable. But, just as with all the other extraordinary research strands, smart surfaces will always and only ever work in conjunction with smart cleaning, smart minimization of surgical intervention to reduce wound size, and really smart prescription and use of antibiotics.[126] (Chorus.)

The long second age of antibiotics isn't just about innovation in materials. The long second age is the one where we use the antibiotics we know about as best we can, where shorter courses, more precisely targeted, are going to be the ones that work against infection and limit bacterial resistance. The long second age is where stewards like Esmita continually do the science necessary to optimize how we use what we've already got. They calculate the exact dosage metrics, as well as when to modulate or de-escalate prescription and usage. They strive for precision in identifying what bacteria are doing the infecting, then target the antibacterial against that and prescribe it for the shortest course possible. Stewardship science is searching for ways to stop long before the point-of-last-resort class of antibiotics, for all the obvious reasons. Shortening courses of drugs means shorter stays in hospital, less exposure to hospital-based infections. Patients can't get *Acinetobacter baumannii* from a hospital bed rail if they aren't holding on to it in the first place.

New antibiotics, used with the same cautious precision, would be good. But we haven't found any new antibiotic classes in the first two decades of the twenty-first century, so a better option is old antibiotics that we rediscover and add to the therapeutic armamentarium as if they were new, and use as carefully as, well, a newborn antibiotic. For humans to search for existing antibiotic compounds would be difficult and second-age time-consuming. Far better to develop an algorithm that allows the artificial intelligence of a computer to do the work for them (the technical term for this is computational chemoinformatics, but AI will do). And so far, this seems to be working. During 2019, scientists at the Massachusetts Institute of Technology in the United States trained the neural network of a computer to search across all the chemical libraries it could find to suggest molecules that might have antibacterial powers we had not realized. In the helpfully (hopefully) named Drug Repurposing Hub, among 107 million others, they found one. Halicin was in the chemical library because its molecules had once been thought useful in the treatment of diabetes, so compounds that used them had gone through trials and toxicity protocols. Halicin has a surprisingly easy-to-read antibiotic chemical name (perhaps because it was given it by computer scientists, not microbiologists, who named it for Hal, the artificial intelligence at the heart of the film *2001: A Space Odyssey*). Once identified, scientists tested it against the worst kinds of resistant bacteria. In each case (in each petri dish, and then in live animal testing), halicin prevented the development of resistance and destroyed the bacterial strain – from *E. coli*, even up to *Acinetobacter baumannii*[127] – which makes it the rarest of things: a rediscovered, effective broad-spectrum antibiotic. And halicin's resistance frequency is low, which means it doesn't learn resistance quickly, so, potentially, it can keep on working for a good while longer.

AI isn't magic, but it saves a great deal of time and broadens our options. Bacteria can still learn resistance – *will* still learn resistance (because they've got apps for that). We'll need to make sure we use the newly rediscovered drugs as carefully as possible. AI is fast, thorough, and only as good as the humans who define its analytic starting points; we need to make sure that we are setting the right parameters for AI, because it's easy to assume that all patients, all over the world, are the same, and that bias then becomes part of the search infrastructure. We have a way to go in properly and fully representing all the different kinds, races, genders and ages of humans who suffer and need remedies for their suffering – something for the programmers of deep-learning machines and intelligences to bear in mind. If they want some help, they should be including stewards in the process of defining search algorithms, and helping the machines themselves to learn. Stewards enable properly participatory AI – more about that in the next chapter, in an unexpected research site, up in the Andes (pack a jumper).

To truly understand how whole sections of the human population can get left out of research processes, we should focus on the most vulnerable population in the world to resistant bacterial infections: children under five years old. Children's immunity to infection can be primed to fail for a number of reasons. They may be malnourished, or their mother may be malnourished, or they may be cold when they should be kept warm. Pregnant women often get urinary tract infections, and if it is a resistant strain, the pathogen gets passed on to the child, in all its resistivity. If a child is born in hospital, no matter how careful their carers are, they can get resistant bacterial infections from the equipment that interfaces with their living tissue, just like adults on critical care wards – tubes and catheters, taking the resistant bacteria straight to where they want to go. Or infection can come from something simpler, like a breast-milk pump. And if newborns get infections, then they are much more likely to get sepsis. Sepsis is the body's own extreme reaction to an infection – not an infection in itself, but something much worse, much worse, much more deadly. In 2018, three million children all over the world got sepsis, and 214,000 of those died.[128] What a terrible waste of human potential. When medical scientists use the phrase 'huge burden of disease', nowhere does it apply more readily and devastatingly than to neonatal sepsis. Forty per cent of bacterial infections likely to cause sepsis are resistant to the combination of antibiotics that are recommended by the current WHO guidelines, yet the guidelines are the only thing medics have, and the boxes of guideline-recommended tablets are the only thing they can offer a family with a very sick child, so they keep on prescribing them, and, increasingly, children keep shivering as sepsis tightens its grip.

Despite this huge burden of disease, there is almost no paediatric-specific antimicrobial resistance research. There are almost forty new antibiotics currently being developed, but only two are for use in children. There would be none at all if it wasn't for the Global Antibiotic Research and Development Partnership (GARDP). GARDP was initiated by the WHO in 2019 and brings together everyone with expertise in the field, from stewards to scientists to the pharmaceutical and biotechnology industries. GARDP is aiming to develop five new antibiotics by 2025, at least two of which will be paediatric specific. It is also working on neonatal sepsis, the breaker of families. The work has started with the biggest study of neonatal sepsis ever done: 3,000 children. It's difficult and complicated and emotional to do trials involving children, and this alone can put researchers off. So this is a miraculously large number for a study of sick children, and it proves, as much as anything else, that it can be done. It's a new, durable line against the Horseman, running around the world, from places like Kilifi Hospital in Kenya to St George's Hospital, Tooting, in the UK. When it is published (about the same time as this book), we will know more about the condition than we ever have before. It will create a solid evidence base, an infrastructure for how we think about paediatric sepsis in the future.

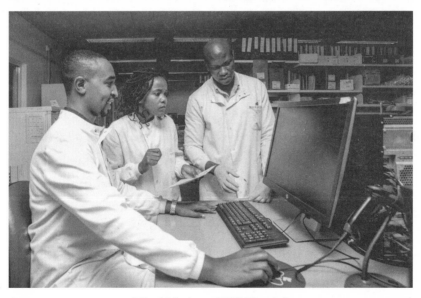

Microbiologists at Kilifi Hospital,
researching the fosfomycin trial data, May 2020.

At the same time, at Kilifi Hospital, they are trialling a different antibiotic therapy for the condition from the one currently recommended in the guidelines (ampicillin-gentamicin). Not new, just different. A new combination of drugs we already know about, but hadn't used before for children (fosfomycin and amikacin). So it's like the halicin discovery, but on a much smaller scale, and the intelligence is purely human. The trial has been a very stewardly one of dosages, timescales and monitoring, and it has kept going throughout the COVID pandemic; the only component that has really slowed down is the submission process of the articles containing their findings to academic journals. In the meantime, stepping up to the line against the rider of the white horse are microbiologists and nurses, and the families of the sick babies, who were approached to participate in the study at a time of almost unimaginable personal crisis, and who were able to listen to the request of the researchers and hear them all the way to the end of the question, and understand that this was something new, that might not work, but if it did, there would be far fewer families enduring what they were enduring at that moment. Lines against Horsemen are built with reports, and with the people who grow practised at asking difficult questions of humans in dreadful conditions, in the ruins of a city or the waiting room of a neonatal ICU, and are able to make sense of their answers so things will get better eventually.

And the line is holding really fast and strong, because the Kilifi trial has worked. The new combination of different old drugs is effective and safe against neonatal sepsis. Next comes an even bigger trial, based on the Kilifi figures, to see if the same findings are possible elsewhere in the world, because we always need to bear in mind the geographical particularities of resistance. Then comes the really hard work, across the world. The WHO will need to take a lead in issuing new treatment guidelines, along with training staff to use the medication carefully, increasing public awareness of the change, and getting the drugs manufactured, with new labels on the boxes, and then distributed. Millions of children at risk of sepsis, now and in the future, are waiting, but we are getting there. All of this is also relevant for the rediscovered class of antibiotics, such as halicin. Stewards will remind everyone of the most important message in all of this: don't waste the new (old/different) drugs. Use them in the best way possible, to minimize and delay the development of resistance. We're aiming for a long second age, not a quick turnover.

Finally, there's one thing that we already do today that we know really works: vaccinations. Routine vaccinations are provided by national governments, humanitarian and philanthropic organizations, and (most of them) by the WHO. The vaccinations programmes cover pneumonia, measles, tuberculosis, polio, cholera and diarrhoea.* Since 2000, worldwide deaths from vaccine-preventable diseases have fallen by 70 per cent. It stands to reason that, if children don't get diseases in the first place, then they don't get the complications of those diseases that might require antibiotic treatment. And now

---

* Using vaccinations, polio has been all but expunged from our planet. Wild polio, a cousin, and tricksy when it comes to prevention, was declared eradicated from Africa on 25 August 2020.

we have the numbers that support this, from the epidemiologists and computational biologists that we have all grown used to hearing from recently. They've been working on this for a long time, analysing figures from 2006–18. They studied two vaccines in particular: the pneumonia jab (or, as it is more scientifically known, the pneumococcal vaccine), which also protects against sepsis and meningitis, and the rotavirus vaccine, which protects against diarrhoea. The pneumonia jab saved 23.8 million episodes of illness that would otherwise have been treated with antibiotics. The rotavirus vaccine saved 13.6 million episodes of illness that would otherwise have been treated with antibiotics. So that's 37.4 million doses of antibiotics saved, most of which would not only have been ineffective against disease, but would have greatly and speedily increased the burden of resistance among the world's population of under-fives – the population that can least afford to have it so.[129]

That's without having achieved the universal vaccination targets set in 2000. There were twenty million children in our world who, in 2018, were under-vaccinated – some had some of the right vaccinations, some had none at all. Vaccination rates during 2020 fell significantly in the early stages of the global pandemic because staff were needed elsewhere and no one quite knew how the system was going to work. Gaps opened up, and we know who loves to ride through a gap. But they didn't stay open for long. When the lists were compiled of essential medical provisions that had to continue no matter what, childhood vaccinations were on them. National healthcare systems that had the capacity picked up their vaccination programmes where they left off. Medical staff from the WHO, from

UNICEF, from the Gates Foundation went to the populations who needed vaccinations with mobile outreach teams, often working in the open air (better than a socially distanced medical-centre waiting room). These were five-day vaccination epics, hundreds of thousands of children inoculated, jabs or oral doses, one after the other, while being held in the arms of their masked family members or carers. Drive-through vaccination clinics were constructed where it was possible, and where it was not, vaccinators went door to door, school to school, boat to boat, tent to tent in refugee camps, stepping back when a response came to their call and speaking clearly through their PPE, explaining what they were there for. And this was not firefighting – this was vaccination as it is normally done, in an ideal world, with record keeping, short questionnaires asking what jabs or drops the child had already had, and explanations of what they needed to come back for. Plans were made for catch-up and follow-up (and a little COVID guidance along the way).[130] We don't yet know when 2020 got back to 2018 levels (or maybe even a bit better), but we know that, when the question was asked about priorities during the pandemic, after a deep breath, the answer from national governments, international non-governmental organizations and the WHO came back loud and clear: vaccinate, no matter what.

It's easy to hold the line when the footholds are well-designed vaccinations in programmes that are already tested and proven, with vaccinators that are trusted, and now with figures that show all of it works even better than we'd ever hoped, better than magic. All stewards know that it isn't actually antibiotics that are healthcare systems by other means, it's vaccinations. The rest of us have come to understand that the priority should always be getting the vaccine, in whatever form it comes in, to those who need it most and have not had it yet. Lives will be saved, futures saved, and people will be able to live through the long second age of antibiotics, and maybe one day contribute to whatever the third age hopefully becomes. All the babies vaccinated together, a true harvest for the world.[131]

As the line reassembles, there's a good deal of squeezing up to make room for a group almost everyone had given up on. Until 2020, researchers had despaired of the industrial pharmaceutical sector's ability to make a viable contribution to a solution to antimicrobial resistance. Resistance in the microbiological world was matched by resistance in the human capitalist marketplace. Pharmaceuticals could make no money developing new antibiotics, so they didn't. There were attempts to address the failure, of which the creation of the GARDP alliance is the most significant, but much of the rest came in global reports, international conferences, calls to action, follow-up reports, more global leadership panels. All they proved really was that there was too much talk and not enough progress, and that, no matter how hard we try, resistant bacterial pathogens cannot be bored to death.[132] But everything is different now. Governments all over the world, researchers and pharmaceutical companies have come together to produce COVID vaccines, and treatments for viral effects and secondary bacterial infections, no matter what the economics are or will be.[133] Pharmaceutical companies don't have to do some of the things that really frightened their risk management and legal teams – like testing drugs on tiny children – because things like the GARDP-led neonatal sepsis study have done the hard, brave work for them. The whole structure – from testing, to intellectual property, to healthcare purchasing systems – is being reorganized, as it should have been a long time ago. After the pandemic is, carefully, declared over, it's back to securing the future for antimicrobial resistance therapeutic R & D, this time with the emphasis on the D.

But we aren't there yet. The tricky bit will be for everyone to remember that what we are working towards is a very long second age of antibiotics. There will be no single point or single year where everything changes, where victory is declared and antimicrobial resistance is vanquished. There is no more magic, as there never really was in the first age, either. As one 2020 commentator reminded us, via the *New England Journal of Medicine*: 'Deaths associated with antibiotic resistance are unlikely to fall to zero . . .'[134] For each new antibiotic we discover, no matter how careful and stewardly we are, no matter how low its resistance frequency is, eventually it will also develop resistance, because nature won't let us have one without the other. So then we will need another new antibiotic, and the participatory AI machines will keep combing the chemical libraries, and the stewards will keep honing their prescription recommendations, and everyone working on everything else that minimizes the exposure of people and hospitals to opportunistic bacterial pathogens will keep on doing their research.

There is no victory over antimicrobial resistance to fight for.[135] Any good steward or professor of infectious diseases will tell you that this is the wrong language, and language can be a deadly distraction. We are playing for a draw. Everyone who holds the line against Pestilence is seeking the most productive draw possible, one that can be continually renegotiated. A dynamic draw is good enough to discourage the rider on the white horse, to get him to put his weapons away and back off. And if he turns to look for the end of the second age, to a time when he is able to reassert his power and take aim at us once more, that point won't be visible on the horizon of our world, not for a good long while.

FAMINE

'. . . and lo a black horse; and he that sat on him had a pair of balances in his hand.'

Revelation 6:5

While Pestilence draws his power from the microbiological world – bacteria, viruses and other one-celled beings called protozoa (which cause the burden of diseases such as malaria) – he doesn't claim it all for himself. The Horsemen do their best work together because they are always prepared to share. So, one significant component of the microbiological world belongs to the rider of the black horse: the fungi. As far as we know (and we know enough to know that's not very far), there are six million separate species of fungi. Most of them live symbiotically or mutually, alongside or as part of other living things. Sometimes, this symbiosis does no harm to host organisms. Often, it is of mutual benefit.[136] But not all species are this considerate, and these fungi are the ones that most interest the rider of the black horse, because it is through them that human beings can not only be infected with disease, they can be made to starve.

Of those six million, 8,000 fungal species are parasitic or pathogenic (disease-causing). Many of them follow a plant-based diet and
when they identify a species that suit them, they invade the living
organism, destroy its defences and feed on the nutrients contained in
its cells – nutrients that other living creatures, like us, for instance,
might otherwise eat. Sometimes, when the fungi have finished, they
leave the plant damaged, vulnerable to diseases, but somehow alive,
but most times all that is left is field after field of dead, empty husks.
Find, feed, kill, move on. No wonder fungi have got their own
Horseman overseeing this process; fungi destroys 20 per cent of the
entire world's food crops each year. Then, another 10 per cent are
lost to different fungal pathogens after harvest, in storage or during
distribution.[137] No drought, hell or high water. Just pathogenic fungi
getting to our food supply and making it theirs, leaving much less
for us. The greatest wastage of food happens where crops are grown,
wherever in the world we grow them. A third of everything we need
to eat is gone before most of us knew it was under threat.[138] And
this is a very old kind of threat, one that evolved an aeon before we
did, hungrier than us, and more patient.

We muddle up our understanding of fungi by thinking they are
plants, because the fungi we can most easily see grow alongside or on
plants. But most biologists are beginning to think that fungi are more
closely related to animals than plants. Other biologists think this is
animal bias – animal-centred science: how typically human. But the
easiest thing to remember is that fungi have their own kingdom.[139]
Animal kingdom, plant kingdom, fungal kingdom. Bacteria have their
own kingdom too, but viruses haven't, because they aren't living

things, and only living things can be awarded their own kingdom (by biologists, who study living organisms). Fungi haven't just been awarded a kingdom – we've also given them their own age. The age of the fungi, when fungi ruled the world. It occurred about 500 million years ago and it lasted around forty million years. The fungi who ruled it looked the part. Some of them were huge, up to a metre across and several metres high – almost theatrically large, just as we might imagine giant fungi to be, but real, and covering the planet.

There's a fossil record for this age, and initially we identified the fossils as those of big strange trees, but now we know them to be fungi. They weren't all enormous. Some were what we would now recognize as mushrooms, and we find them preserved in Jurassic amber. Some were water moulds or downy mildews, a few fine layers thick. Some were almost invisible, and we call them microfossils, and they are the very oldest fossils of all. Getting fungal origin stories sorted out is important, because – this is why research money is piling in – a fossil record that accounts for non-plant/animal life forms may be useful when we go exploring on Mars. Just as with biofilm fossils, if we recognize that strange formations in other planets' sedimentary layers could be fungal in origin, then we might have a better sense of how life is happening there, based on what we already know happened here.[140]

In the age of the fungi, the days were long (eighteen hours of light) and there was good eating to be found from the previous two billion years' worth of debris from the very simple life forms that preceded the fungi (mostly bacterial biofilms that had bubbled up on the prebiotic soup).[141] As the biggest living organisms on Earth, fungi dominated their age. Not just because of their size or numbers, but because of their extraordinary, pioneering resilience. The age of the fungi survived asteroid strikes, volcanic eruptions and ice ages – six, possibly seven separate extinction-level events that struck the planet. Fungi adapted, strengthened, shrank almost to invisibility, but endured. Over time, forty million years of it, fungi have come to understand what the rules are to ensure for a successful species with its own kingdom. Rule One: cooperate with species from other kingdoms. Rule Two: but only ever on your own terms. Rule Three: when cooperation no longer nourishes sufficiently, compete aggressively.

What and how they eat is what makes them fungi. To support their own cells, they need to eat preformed organic compounds – something that already comes in a food form, which is why so many of them prefer a plant-based meal.[142] Although, fungi eating is really eating by other means. Fungi don't have digestive capabilities or the ability to make their own food by photosynthesis (so they truly, definitely are not plants). Instead, they release a powerful enzyme that breaks down the cell walls of whatever material they are living on (or in), so they can get at and absorb its nutrients. The enzymes fungi produce are capable of processing material as tough and thick as bone and bark, slowly (not always), but surely. Some fungi will only eat crap, in the form of dying or dead or excreted organic material, and only fungi can recycle organic matter in this way naturally. Scale it up, across the planet, through the ages, and it's this process that creates the soil in which we grow food. We live in and by the space their eating creates. If the fungi that rot (eat) trees didn't exist, we'd have been overwhelmed by forests long ago.

If they are getting enough to eat, fungi spread by producing spores, mostly from their wispy ends (hyphae). Some do this asexually, and some have fungi sex, which can be observed under microscopes, and many mycologists (fungi specialists) spend a great deal of time watching this and describing it: 'Anybody who has watched a chytrid zoospore crawling like an amoeba along the body of a nematode searching for the best site to encyst, and then winding in its flagellum, encysting and penetrating the host will never forget the experience. All these events can be followed in simple glass chambers on microscope slides.'[143]

If fungi were to fill out a personality test, they would probably say that their three favourite things are eating, warm weather and travel, and their most positive trait is their resilience. So if there is no warm weather, they can overwinter. They can endure unseasonably long periods of cold or drought. They can survive unexpected changes in the composition of the materials they've been living in, so if things suddenly get saltier, for instance, or more radioactive, they adapt. For a long while, to travel, they had to wait for the right wind, but when it blew, on they hopped, and they were carried across continents. As humans learned to harness the wind for their huge sailing ships to carry agricultural cargoes across oceans, fungi stowed away, and this new form of transportation was much more frequent and regular, and increasingly obliging, as sail gave way to steam and oil-fired power.

This is how fungal pathogens travel, live and work, in their most aggressive form. In the mid-nineteenth century, a fungal pathogen that ate potatoes arrived in Europe from South America. It came in clipper ships that took the long way round, from the Pacific coast to the North Atlantic shores, carrying guano (bird-crap fertilizer) and potato plants. There may have been fungi in the crap, but more likely it was already in the plants, making not much of a living eating potatoes that grew at high altitudes and generally tolerated the fungi's best efforts in a sort of truce. When the plants arrived in Europe, where the weather was warmer, the climate was wetter and the fields were only a few metres above sea level, the potato fungus realized that the terms of the truce no longer applied, and it could feast.

The first signs of blight were large black spots on mature potato-plant leaves, which gradually spread to the tuber, rotting it like gangrene. When the fungus had finished, what was left of the potato was inedible and economically useless. If they could afford it, farmers all over Europe tried to strengthen their fields before they reseeded by adding fertilizer, but this only made things worse. Crops came back more quickly, initially stronger, but providing even richer food for fungi, which grew stronger still, over and over again. The destruction of a vital staple crop, occurring against a background of human society already sick from economic causes, led to famine. In Ireland, where the first large-scale infestation was reported in 1845, potato blight spread faster than cholera, and killed more viciously, family after family. Three million people either starved or were forced into migration, nothing left of their families but the paupers' graves in the churchyards, nothing left of the life they had known but the endless fields of rotting tubers.

By 1852, what had now been called the Great Famine was over. The few remaining Irish farmers who clung to their land had switched to other crops, or pasture for livestock. Potato blight only eats potato, so it in turn starved and was much diminished. The black horse galloped away, because there was nothing more for his rider to do, nothing left to take, but not because humans had held a line against him. There was no line for them to hold. All their assumptions about potato blight were muddled up and wrong, for deep, non-scientific reasons. Fungi, especially the species forms it takes that we can see, have strong mythological associations with death and decay. Some fungi (the saprotrophs) do live off dying or dead plants, but not all. Myth is bad on details like that, and shapes science more than we'd like to admit. Nineteenth-century scientists thought the potato plant had a disease and that it was dying when the fungus took hold, that the fungi were there cleaning up the dead, as they always did, as they all did. So, all the science was directed to holding a line against a bacterial disease that wasn't there.[144] For decades, they misread the sign of the black spot on leaves as meaning the aftermath of disease. It didn't. It meant a fungus had taken hold of a completely healthy plant – a fungus that was invisible during the early, infectious stages. It was not cooperating with the potato plant, not negotiating terms, but competing aggressively, and winning. Potato blight is not a saprotroph, it is a biotroph – a fungus that needs a living subject, that will not be happy with a dead or dying one.

If the nineteenth-century scientists weren't able to hold the line in their own time, they would eventually contribute to its strengthening in the future. From the first year of the famine, scientists had collected and preserved samples of the diseased potato plants: their leaves, slices of tuber and seeds. The horror of the famine, and of future famines, meant they did this conscientiously and carefully – and quickly, because if left too long, the sample plant material would discolour, and the black spots would no longer be obvious against the remaining healthy leaf tissue when future researchers came to look at them. Leaves, stems, roots and tubers were gathered and pressed flat on to absorbent paper, a label inscribed on the page with dates and names and places of where they had been found. Then, the pages of absorbent paper were bound together and sent to botanical collections for storage, preservation and the generation of hope. As the samples were assembled all over the world, scientists gradually realized the true microbiological nature of what they were dealing with, and new branches of natural sciences were born, properly focused on fungi as pathogens, not just symptoms or death throes. Improvements in microscope technology meant scientists could now see the previously invisible fungi world, in all its strange detail. It would be a while before they would have cameras to capture images of this new world, but in the meantime, they could draw what they saw through their lenses, and print what they drew, with extraordinary skill. Across the world, a new portfolio – a catalogue – of beautiful images of fungi was created. It transformed understanding and created a subject that could be taught to an international standard. Along with the pressed plant-material samples, it was the first systematic list of all the fungi known to humans. Prints remain sharp and resilient and useful (and may do so for longer than digital photographic images).

So, while science began the process of understanding, fungi, who had never had any doubt as to their essential nature, endured. Potato blight may have been starved into submission in Ireland, but it never disappeared entirely. A few spores were still living dormant in quiescent survival, but always waiting. Black spots appeared on potato crops in smallholdings, or in people's vegetable gardens, although not with the same impact as the mid-century's infestation. When it came back, it was recognized for what it was, and efforts began to combat it. Old and new chemical treatments were applied, but above all, scientists sought to breed out the weakness that allowed the blight to flourish, by crossing the seeds from one flowering potato plant, which cropped well and tasted good, with another, which was known to be resilient, and hoping that the resulting seeds would be stronger than their parents. And then they waited, for two seasons, because selective breeding of potatoes takes much longer than for most other plants.

We've always done selective breeding, whether as farmers, gardeners or scientists. We cross plants with desirable characteristics to produce something new and improved. It speaks to a very old yearning to reach for somewhere in the biosphere where there are botanical Platonic ideals – perfect forms of plants, combining the strength of wild nature and the richness of human agronomy. Paradise is always a cultivated garden, and there are no Horsemen in Eden. Selective breeding underpins our cultivation and domestication of all living things, from pedigree dogs to prize-winning orchids, and potatoes.* Each time new potato tubers were successfully bred and formed, everyone dared to hope they would be perfect and that Famine would be banished back to where it came from and know its place. In 1939, a new blight-proof potato hybrid was triumphantly shown at the Chelsea Flower Show in London, alongside the selectively bred roses and new sweet-pea varieties. Farmers sowed the seed plants in field trials with some success and then took them to their farms and waited for the first shoots. Just as it had done with all the previous attempts, the blight came back, sharpened its teeth on the new version, and wiped out the main crop.

In the meantime, apart from selective breeding, the weapon we have used most consistently against fungal pathogens (or whatever we thought they were) is chemical. From organic mixtures made up on farms, to huge factories producing inorganic compounds in plastic bottles, we use fungicides to kill fungi, and sometimes we use fungistatics that halt fungi in their tracks without necessarily killing them. We apply fungicides in powder or liquid forms, from spray-nozzle bottles, from buckets on our backs, from aircraft flying over fields or from expensive agricultural machinery with special attachments and huge tanks for the chemicals. We use chemical fungicides to treat the seeds and seedlings before we plant them (sometimes we heat the seeds to kill spores – known technically as differential

---

* While scientists desperately sought to breed a blight-proof, famine-proof potato, around 1900, in private walled vegetable gardens, private plant enthusiasts cross-bred a variety they named 'Salad Blue', where the leaves were variegated with dark brown patches on the green. They were thought to be very pretty, with bright blue flowers in abundance and blue-stained tubers (best used for roasting, rather than actual salads), and are still popular and still easy to confuse with a blighted potato strain.

thermal sterilization of seed grain). We treat their roots, and the soil around them. Antifungals are applied to fields before the fungus comes, to protect the crop, and after it has arrived, to beat it back. We use them in storehouses, where fungi feed on harvested crops – a huge problem for everyone who farms onions. Onions get all kinds of fungal pathogens while they are moved from field to kitchen – black mould, blue mould, grey rot, soft rot, smudge rot and, most dreaded of all, neck rot. Think about how often we use onions, how we expect them to be available all year round. This means storage, at just the right temperature and just the right humidity, and it means spraying them with sulphur treatments to kill the fungi that would otherwise destroy the stored crop. There might be a more sustainable solution, where essential oils of thyme are used instead of sulphur on the huge warehouses of onions around the world, but it will only ever be temporary.

Because, just like bacteria in the face of antibacterials, fungi are smart and metabolically versatile. They have had all the time in the world to learn to adapt. The fungi at the Chernobyl nuclear power plant site survived – even flourished – after the catastrophe in 1986.[145] Biologists from Ukraine and around the world have been into the exclusion zone to take samples. Searching for fungi has always been a dangerous business, whether it's climbing into the high, freezing Andes to hunt for disease signs on plants or working in the aftermath of the world's worst nuclear accident. To get their samples from Chernobyl, the biologists had to wear the heaviest of hazmat suits, with built-in respirator units, allowing for only short periods of exploration during which they had to be careful not to trip up in the heavy steel-toed boots necessary to prevent ground-based contamination coming up through their feet. And when they took all this off and looked at their samples, they found that fungi have adapted their wispy end bits (the hyphae) not only to counteract the effects of ionizing radiation, but also to resist the effects of the increasingly frequent fires in the region. There is something that might be evidence that fungi are perhaps even absorbing radiation from the plentiful plant debris they are feeding off. In the wildest dreams of scientists, we might somehow use fungi to clean up contaminated radioactive sites, although on the flipside of wildest dreams are easily conjured nightmares, where fungi, juiced up on radioactive isotopes, think it's time to begin the second age of the fungi.

While fungi are almost infinitely versatile, our model for combatting them using chemicals is distinctly unversatile. In the agrochemical business, fungicides are usually 'single-target site' formulations, targeting only one process in the fungal activities of daily life. Most of them work by preventing the fungus from building up the protective membranes and boundaries of its cells, so it can't produce the enzymes needed to eat its food. But, just like bacteria, whatever we try to kill fungi with, we never quite get them all; there are always a few left dormant, waiting. They learn and adapt, proving that, eventually, whatever doesn't kill you makes you stronger next time round. We certainly know by now we can't fungicide our way to a new Eden. Today, 15 per cent of all global fungicide sales are to combat potato blight.

And this is despite our finally having a good (but not full) sense of exactly what kind of biotroph the potato-blight fungus is. Genetic sequencing can not only give us the DNA of today's living organisms, it can also trace their history and family lineage, provided the samples are good enough to retain sufficient genetic material to be analysed.[146] The twenty-first-century scientists who set out to do this forensic microbiology went back in time to the original catalogues and found plenty of good samples pressed into the absorbent paper and carefully labelled by their collectors. After what must have been forests of forms to fill in, they were able to extract viable samples from 186 leaves that clearly showed the black spot of blight and that had been carefully stored in herbariums and natural history collections, waiting for just this moment to tell their story, finally.

In 2004, the DNA results were published. Eighty-six per cent of all the herbarium specimens from historical outbreaks across the world were infected with the same fungal pathogen.[147] As they sequenced each sample, the scientists could trace the blight as it developed and travelled around the world, and they found it had been more widely dispersed than originally thought. Small differences could be discerned – a few haplotypes' worth (a haplotype is a group of genes within an organism that was inherited together from a single parent). But each one provided clear evidence of the small but crucial steps taken by the fungi to adapt to specific environments – temperature, rainfall, altitude, chemicals – working out how to live with the new conditions and then off them. Similar techniques were used in 2020 to trace the spread of COVID-19 around the world, with scientists noting the small genetic mutations, step by step, patient by patient, because this is how we do things now. But the complete journey can be seen in the identification of the potato-blight fungal family, which, with all its little haplotype variants, has a name: *Phytophthora infestans* (which translates, perhaps a bit unexcitingly, as 'plant-borne infester'). *Phytophthora infestans* is every haplotype as dangerous as it was in 1845. The last really catastrophic blight event in the USA occurred in 1992. There was a significant outbreak in 2009, and individual cases have been reported all over European production fields in 2020.[148] It's still going, still competing.*

DNA sequencing is cataloguing by the most modern of means, and cataloguing, no matter when it happens, is an act of preservation, of science and of hope. Every scientist who thought to keep the diseased leaves of dying plants that they didn't really understand, who did their job so well, without fridges or bright lights, so that each leaf they preserved had its DNA laboratory-standard intact, all of them were investing in a future solution, beyond their time, so that famine would become history. The list of samples used by the twenty-first-century scientists is long, but here are just a few entries,

---

* If you are reading this and you are a mycologist, then you'll have already cried out in anguish: '*Phytophthora infestans* isn't pure fungi, it's an OOMYCETE!' It is, but if you aren't a mycologist, the differences between fungi and oomycetes (pronounced oooh-my-seats) are small and technical, and something we non-mycologists are allowed to muddle up, unproblematically. Oomycetes belong to the algae family, which doesn't have a kingdom of its own. Vaulting ambition has led the oomycetes to seek membership of the fungal kingdom, by becoming more like fungi every day. They do this, haplotype by haplotype, by altering themselves at the genetic level to eat like fungi, reproduce like fungi, travel like fungi, compete like fungi. They have nothing to prove to their Horseman when it comes to making human beings starve. Twenty per cent of oomycete DNA now looks like its fungal equivalent. We'll watch them transform in real time, via our sequencers. But, for all intents and purposes, in this book, they are the same.

showing how international and serious and sustained the effort to find a solution for blight was:

Year	Collector	Country
1845	M. Desmazieres	France
1866	P. A. Karsten	Finland
1875	J. E. Vize	England
1880	W. Trelease	USA
1889	P. Hennings	Chile
1897	S. Rostowzew	Russia

Their pressings were added to collections housed in the mycological sections of the herbariums, from the Royal Botanic Gardens at Kew to the USDA National Fungus Collection in Beltsville, Maryland, and the Museum of Evolutionary Botany in Uppsala, Sweden. Today, we can add to the list the names of the mycologists – the closest thing to superstars they have in mycology – who did the forensic genetics that built on the work of their forerunners: K. J. May and J. B. Ristaino, North Carolina State University, 2004.[149] And they could only do it with authority because the samples from the nineteenth century had been treated with such respect and hope by the collections in which they were housed.

Even so, everywhere, funding for botanical gardens and national plant collections is being cut. So, if you want to join the line easily and with great benefits, get an annual membership to the one nearest your home. They are always beautiful places to visit, especially for those of us that live in cities and don't have gardens of our own, and, when they reopened after the pandemic confinements, they were quiet green blessings. Beyond the gift shops and public engagements are the labs where the work is done, where the low hum of air conditioning controls the temperature of samples, going back, and hopefully forward, for centuries, as a resource. What nineteenth-century pressed plant samples were to the forensic biologists in 2004, the DNA sequence catalogues will be to those using artificial intelligence (AI) search strategies in the (not too distant) future. It's all the same thing, really. People looking carefully. The National Botanic Gardens in Dublin, Ireland are wonderful, and it's particularly meaningful that their website contains useful information on how to press plant samples correctly, and what kind of information to include on the label if it is to be useful to future generations.[150] It's surprising what we still have yet to sample. Somewhere along the way, in the first age of antibiotics, we forgot to sample Fleming's original *Penicillium* mould. In July 2020, we finally did it. We haven't done anything with what we now know, just yet, but this is one gene sequence that is as pleasing to historians as it is to microbiologists and mycologists.[151]

There would have been potatoes in Eden, and we know there have been potatoes in our world for at least 8,000 years, sustaining the earliest humans. For some of us, potatoes are a side dish – the carbohydrate that soaks up sauce, or the finger-friendly chips that are easy and wonderful to eat. But, for much of the world, they are a whole lot more than that. Potatoes are the third most important global crop, in terms of human consumption. They are good, nutritious eating, providing lots of protein and carbohydrate, and they are an excellent economic crop (hence the magnitude of the catastrophe when they failed in Ireland, in 1845). They crop more than once a year, and tubers can grow as big as their surroundings will let them, without damaging their parent plant (wheat and rice stalks can only bear so much weight before collapsing). The first potato plants grew in the Andes – not down at the foot, where you might expect plants to come from, but higher up, between 3,000 and 5,000 metres above sea level. Up where the air is clear, because it's thin from lack of oxygen, and where it's dry, because any water from the plant or soil surface evaporates quickly, and where the temperatures drop to frigid each night, most of the year round. The soil is tough on the higher slopes of the Andes, and the land gradients are steep, so the roots of any plants that grow there have their work cut out for them clinging to the hillside. Four thousand separate potato varieties worked out how to survive on the mountainsides and were tough enough to make it into our time. Some need shredding and drying before they are edible, but some are so sweet the locals who farm them eat them for elevenses with their coffee or hot chocolate.

The 4,000 varieties had some help from humans along the way. Over time, Andean farmers worked out how to manage this almost vertical agricultural space, using very small, intricate canal systems that they carved out of the mountainsides to cascade water from high points to low, irrigating the fields in between.[152] They had centuries to work the system out, to build a line and hold it. When the potatoes failed, the earliest farmers and their families starved, but as they discovered plants that made it through the winter and didn't mind the frost, everyone flourished, and seeded and grew. Around them, also from the mountains and built on this heritage, grew an entire empire. The Inca state formally owned all the land of its domain, and those who farmed it received part of their crop for themselves and their family, and the rest went to central stores for use by the officers of state, or for redistribution in times of food insecurity. The Inca state also harvested the labour of the farmers in the off season, moving them around the empire to build huge cities, roads and hydraulic networks.

The Inca state existed because of the learning done over centuries of farming and living in the mountains. They didn't waste any of it. Its inspectors kept accounts of productivity and crop yields, passing them through the central administration to its cadre of agricultural researchers and scientists, who worked to increase food supplies and security so the empire could continue to grow. The high point of the convergence of farming heritage and Inca state-building came sometime in the fifteenth century, when labouring farmers built the extraordinary site of Moray, in modern-day Peru, for their imperial masters. Moray is sometimes called the 'Inca Agricultural College' – although scientists now think it is more likely to have been an experimental agricultural station, state-owned and run, and therefore built grandly, much like the Victorian public buildings in Britain whose scale and architectural features reflected the importance of their work for the whole empire. Architects and builders of the Inca adapted existing sinkholes to create a series of circular terraces. In each of the walled terraces, fields were cultivated that had separate soil, temperature, altitude and rainfall features (technically called whatever the Inca phrase was for ecoclimatic equivalence class sectors). They would have tried out crops such as maize, quinoa and potatoes to see what did best where, and what their tolerance levels were. The intricate canal systems were adapted from those used by the farmers around the empire, and they allowed the water supply to be controlled as part of the testing. The Incas may also have used complex cosmological measurements to determine sowing and production schedules (what today we call biodynamics).

The Moray site isn't ancient, but it represents the culmination of a particularly Andean agricultural format and tradition of agricultural experimentation existing alongside production. No academic silos here, from what the archaeologists can see. From individual farmers, in individual fields, working out which plants grew the best on the high mountain terraces, to a huge state enterprise – everyone was undertaking the same work to make the land produce enough food sustainably. The intensive sustainability that we strive for today is not a recent concept. And then, a century after the Moray experimental site was built, came horsemen and riders – not gods, but colonizers from Europe – who smashed the Inca state, killing much of its population with the pestilence of disease, pushing farmers back to subsistence living in the mountains, and enslaving many of the rest. Everything learned at Moray was lost. The varieties of potatoes in development were rewilded, pushed to the sidelines, scruffy and uncultivated, pulled up as weeds. Centuries passed before pre-colonial knowledge was gradually re-established. With no central authority interested in their work, farmers became stewards of their own small fields, clinging to life on the mountainsides, passing plants and knowledge down precariously through their families, but not much further. In the meantime, because of the demands of its urban population, Peru became an importer of potatoes.

The Andean farmers kept the cultivation of potatoes going long enough for today's scientists to take notice of their stewardship and help them safeguard their gains. Since 1971, they have had the support of the Centro Internacional de la Papa (CIP). The Centro has offices in Peru, Ecuador and Chile. The forensic genetics done in 2004 confirmed that it was potato plants from Ecuador that were exported with such catastrophic consequences in the nineteenth century to places that were low and damp and warm, and that surrendered so easily to blight. Because we still don't live in a blight-free Eden, the Centro's vision is 'a healthy, inclusive and resilient world through root and tuber systems'.[153] Sweet potato and other roots and tubers were added to the mandate of the CIP in 1988, and this was reflected in a redesign of their logo, which shows a pre-Andean farmer in traditional costume, holding a potato plant in one hand and a sweet-potato plant (pointed ends) in the other.* They also work on research that will benefit tomato crops, because it was CIP scientists who worked out that, a very long time ago, potatoes and tomatoes came from the same family, and so the *Phytophthora infestans* affects them both.

---

* Please note a key difference: a sweet potato is not quite the same as a potato, because it's a storage root, not a tuber. A potato is a tuber, which is really a thickened stem.

The office of the CIP has some of the most beautiful research stations in the world, between hills and snow-covered volcanoes, and there are llamas (with their interesting antibody profiles) at the sides of the roads. The air is thin and clear, and on sunny days it makes the sky especially blue. CIP scientists spend most of their time searching for old, wild varieties of potato, whose tough family traits can be woven back into the genome. One of them is agronomist Dr Alberto Salas. Alberto is a legend in the CIP and beyond, and he works with 'an unquenchable thirst to unearth potato wild relatives'. Alberto the potato-scientist-steward has worked for fifty years, wherever potatoes grow wild. It has been a lifelong fascination for him, and he remembers every wild potato species he has ever seen, since he was a child, and where they grew, and he's been on hundreds of field trips to see if they are still there. He is a human catalogue. He knows that potatoes usually grow by rocks, on steep slopes, or under thorny bushes to keep animals like llamas from eating too many of them. He has watched how what used to be footpaths into the mountains, trodden by pre-Incan and Incan farmers, have become tarmac roads, so now wild potatoes often grow right by the roadside. He's spotted them from the windows of buses, and he's paid the driver and the other passengers to stop the bus and wait for him to dash out and dig up the plant, all of them watching him, wondering why this man is bothering with weeds that most people would simply yank out of their fields and throw aside.

Alberto carries a satchel, and a short-handled pick for digging up plants, and huge flower presses in which he uses newspapers for blotting paper, so he can bring samples down the mountain for their germplasm to be extracted and catalogued. He has a phone now, which makes recording locations easier, but there isn't always a signal, so he works with whatever comes to hand. We might think the Horsemen stand a long way off while Alberto works, but in the 1980s, he'd have felt the snorts of the red horse of War close by. Large parts of Peru were under the control of the Shining Path terrorist group, the ISIS of their day. Alberto's potato expeditions often passed through their territory, and he was detained by them five times. But he managed to survive and continue on his way. And he still does today, and is training a new generation to take the line around the world high into the Andes, securing it in altitudes where most of us would struggle to breathe, let alone spot a tiny blue flower that signifies a root-and-tuber system that grows and flourishes in the cold, that has reached an accommodation with its enemies and may one day save us all. By 2020, 60 per cent of all the samples in the CIP gene bank were contributed by Alberto.

When Alberto brings in a new plant specimen to the laboratories of the CIP, it's carefully unpacked and logged into their herbarium and cryopreservation unit, where they keep seed and in vitro samples of leaf and root specimens. Then, gene by gene, each potato plant is catalogued. This is all big potato tech, needing cold, constant temperatures and a lot of power. Just in case, and just as their predecessors did, and because it's the way Alberto does it, they also press leaves and stems into acid-free tissue paper and write a label describing when and where it was sampled. They add QR codes to each, to keep all their options open, and keep them in big boxes at room temperature. This is food security, by other means, the old and the new, enabling us to be safe and sure.

At the CIP, they know what the scientists working to find blight-free potatoes in the twentieth century knew: it is technically very difficult to create completely new potato varieties. It isn't that potatoes don't have very varied genes – they do, many, and each with incredible potential. But their genetic structure is complex, hard to manage and really unpredictable. Genes that aren't supposed to be in the new variety sneak in, no matter how carefully potato plants are cross-bred to produce new seeds. Working out what isn't working is almost impossible until a plant grows and the scientist can see what's actually happening, and can then sequence it to see where they may have gone wrong. Results take years. Breeding new potato varieties is as difficult as finding a wild potato plant on an Andean mountainside among tangles of weeds if you aren't Alberto Salas. It involves crossing, recrossing, selecting and recombining. Finally, tubers have to be planted and harvested to be tested and reproduced. Elsewhere, commercial potato agronomists are working on developing potato hybrids that have simpler genetic identities, from which they can be more easily and precisely bred. They've planted sentinel test fields of them in the Democratic Republic of the Congo. There's nothing for farmers yet, but there may be, especially once the process is combined with the richness of the CIP's herbarium and cryostorage holdings.[154]

The CIP has been careful and patient. They know their history, so they take a good long view. It's taken decades, but to date the CIP has released eight solid new varieties of potato. The results have strengthened inherent resistance features, reintroducing family lines that go back to Inca times, restoring the genitive diversity strength to fight the blight. CIP potato and sweet-potato varieties are not just resistant, but also more highly nutritious. In 2020, they released a new sweet-potato variety, enriched with vitamin A – the technical term for this kind of plant is a 'nutri-dense crop' – and that doesn't mind drought, provided its farmers are prepared to steward its roots through the dry season.

CIP has always brought local farmers into the line they hold, through its Guardians of the Potato scheme. Just as the Incas did at Moray, CIP scientists are in regular contact with farmers who work at different altitudes and with different soil conditions. The farmers report yields to CIP, and provide data on the traditional techniques they apply and which ones work best. Increasingly, they are tracking the effects of climate change. Their accounts report fewer frosts, later in the year, and how they are moving their fields higher and higher into the mountains to keep up with cold temperatures that in turn keep their crops tough and blight free. In return, CIP is helping them to market, literally. CIP has encouraged small farmers to take their own crops into the cities and sell them as precious and delicious, to be savoured and treasured. They've helped with marketing materials and logos, and really practical things, like producing mesh bags for farmers to use for the long trips down from the mountains to the marketplaces, which are light, and mean the potatoes don't have to be unpacked before they are displayed to customers. Gradually, as with farmers' markets around the world selling heritage food, locals in cities are rediscovering the sheer wonderfulness of native potato varieties, and are prepared to pay a little bit more for them. It helped that CIP also reached out to the most fashionable of Peruvian and Ecuadorian chefs, and the coolest food trucks, inviting them to be part of the process as well. When the pandemic arrived in Peru, CIP was alert to the dangers of transmission in marketplaces, and it has ongoing programmes to help its farmers and their customers keep safe, while maintaining the interest in local production.

CIP might be patient and careful, but it still reaches for the stars beyond the mountains. In 2016, CIP joined a partnership with NASA and the SETI Institute.* If we are to go to other planets, then we will need to be able to grow our own food when we get there, because it won't be possible to take it all with us. In particular, astrobiologists want to find out if there is any way to grow plants on Mars, using soil from the most Mars-like place on Earth: a Peruvian coastal desert which is arid, high altitude, and dotted with closed-basin lakes that used to be full of salty water, leaving behind toxic residues not thought capable of supporting life beyond the bacterial. We think the Gale Crater on Mars may have once looked like this.[155] The soil was taken back to greenhouses at CIP and was planted with a range of crops, including potatoes, beans, corn and carrots. Everything failed, except potatoes. CIP had bred varieties specially to survive the kind of abiotic stress that very salty soil exerts on the plants that try to grow in it, and they endured, and made it through to the next round, and

---

* The mission of the SETI Institute is to explore, understand and explain the origin and nature of life in the universe, and the evolution of intelligence.

the real test. The toughest of them were planted into germination cups, and the cups were placed in soil inside hermetically sealed Martian atmosphere simulators. The simulators were kept at the same temperature and air pressure, with the same levels of light and carbon dioxide as would be found on Mars, and the potatoes grew. THEY GREW. The video feed of the plants growing, leaf by leaf, in real time and real life, is archived on YouTube.[156]

We're a long way from taking potato plants to Mars, never mind growing them, and they'll need watering when they get there. We'll probably need to keep an eye on the fossil findings to see if there are any interplanetary blight ancestors waiting for them, but we know how to do all these things now, on our world. For the CIP, the Potatoes on Mars project has gone a long way towards determining the minimum conditions that a potato can endure to survive, and the real reason we need to know these is not because of imminent space-travel plans, but because of climate change. The varieties that performed so stalwartly in the experiment are now being used by farmers in places on our own planet where what passes for soil grows dryer and saltier and more abiotic every season.[157] The CIP has calculated that five million households across our planet have benefitted from their new potato varieties, which have brought better food, more protein, and are more easily grown by those who have little, whether it's water, soil quality or money to buy fertilizer.[158] The line around the world is especially strong when it runs through the offices and labs of the Centro Internacional de la Papa. Two of its scientists (Hugo Campos and Oscar Ortiz) have compiled the definitive work on the subject – *The Potato Crop: Its Agricultural, Nutritional and Social*

Contribution to Humankind – open access and free to download, for scientists and all potato aficionados.[159]

When the scientists calculate that we lose 20 per cent of all the crops we grow, they are talking about more than potatoes. Just as there are antibacterial stewards, there are also antifungal stewards. The antifungal steward I know best is Professor Sarah Gurr, and her research journey into the line around the world underpins and symbolizes the work to save the planet from the burden borne to us by the rider of the black horse. Sarah was always interested in mycology (the study of fungi). At Imperial College and then Oxford, she studied botany, plant technology and plant pathology. She's been researching fungal plant diseases and their consequences ever since, calling ever more urgently for action to save crops and humans (including in special themed issues of *Philosophical Transactions*). Sarah is currently the professor of food security at the University of Exeter, in Great Britain. She's chosen a hard furrow to plough, but from fungi to fungal pathogens to food security and famine, whatever I've needed to know, I've always started with Sarah. In our very first conversation about fungal crop pathogens, she paused and asked if I had included any material on pressing plants. When I told her I had, she said, 'Good, because researchers and institutions don't do enough pressing, and it's important.' People who press flowers, and label them carefully, join the line.

And then we talked about wheat. When the rider of the black horse had moved off from Ireland, he looked elsewhere for crops to steal and people to starve, and he found our huge modern wheat fields. Wheat contributes a fifth of all that we eat, and it's packed full of protein, starches and carbohydrates. Wheat contains calories that create energy and growth and muscle mass. In the nineteenth century, the crop kept pace with the industrial revolution. It fed its workers, and built empires and created the modern world. This could be done because specialist plant cultivars were introduced and huge new arable systems cleared the earth's natural features and pumped the soil full of fertilizer to make land resource-rich to maximize crop yields for a growing, hard-worked, hungry population. But, in a model that would be repeated in 1940 when bacterials and antibacterials met industrial pharmaceutical production, agriculture scaled up, globalized, industrialized, and the same process was replicated for those organisms, like fungal pathogens, that preyed on what it produced.

Wheat is easy to farm in huge fields, crop after crop, year after year, intensively. Pathogenic fungi that like wheat, and don't want to share it with the humans that grow it, have preyed on it as long as it has been grown. Some don't destroy the crop completely, but they make the flour taste bad (it's why gingerbread was developed in Britain, so that spices covered up the flavour and bakers could make some money in years when bread was scarce). Some reduce the protein content – same wheat, much less nutritious; humans who eat it are full, but not adequately fed – less muscle mass, less energy to work. The most dangerous of all are the wheat rust fungi, which live on the stems and leaves of the plants and leave nothing behind. Wheat rust fungi is easy to spot, no microscope needed, because the leaves or stems of affected plants look like they've begun to rust, like old metal. And rust never sleeps.

Wheat rust fungi defoliate plants before they've had a chance to flower. Nutrients meant for the wheat kernels, and the humans who would otherwise eat them, go instead to the fungus. The stems and roots of the plant don't grow properly. By the time the fungal life-cycle is complete, a field of young green wheat shoots is a tangle of black, ruined stalks. All the rusts produce masses of light, floating spores, and have several cycles of spore production throughout their growing season. Mycologists are quick to reach for a disease analogy, and wheat rust is known as the polio of agriculture – not necessarily because of its speed of transmission, but because of its power. It has multiple varieties, all of them parasitic and destructive. It's wind-borne and is resilient in the transmission stages. It can overwinter, so it damages winter wheat as well as the summer harvest, and it can endure high heat and drought. As it consumes the leaves, their debris provides a kind of rust-specific fertilizer, so the fungi go on eating and reproducing.

Wheat rust fungi are picky but prolific eaters, characterized by their virulence and extreme host specialization. When demand for wheat scales up, so does the fungal pathogen. In 1916, Europe and the United States brought land back into agricultural use to grow wheat to feed the troops fighting the Great War. There was rust, somewhere, waiting. It was one of the worst harvests on record, wheat rust tearing across the acreage on both sides of the Atlantic, and it took years to recover the land through chemical treatment and replanting with different seed varieties. Wheat rust came again in the 1940s, when another world war disrupted food and labour supply, and agricultural patterns. In Mexico, in 1944, a century after *Phytophthora infestans* devastated Ireland, wheat rust halved wheat yields, impoverished farmers and starved their families. The Mexican government, along with the Rockefeller Foundation from the United States, established a Wheat Research and Production programme. On staff was plant pathologist Dr Norman Borlaug, son of Iowan prairie farmers, and obsessed with combatting rust fungus. He began work creating new varieties of wheat that had broad, stable resistance features, adapted well to changing growing conditions and were able to deliver a high yield. Borlaug and his team were able to do this from the get go, producing new varieties that went to farmers all over the world, because wheat, unlike potatoes, is very easy to crossbreed. Features such as sturdy stalks, strong enough to bear heavy heads, fast-growing seeds and less need for long, light days are easy to identify and aim for. Wheat seed is easily generated, stored and transported.[160] For over fifty years, wheat rust and most other types of fungal pathogen were beaten.[161] We discovered a range of fungicides to do it with, naming them the azole class. Azoles are a single-target site fungicide, which only does one thing (break down fungal cell walls), but has been doing it successfully ever since. Wheat yields improved significantly (so we all ate better) and Famine was (mostly) averted. Borlaug was eventually awarded the Nobel Peace Prize, in 1970, because building a line against one Horseman usually ends up holding the rest of them back too.[162]

The period in which agriculture was transformed by new seed types, new fertilizers and fungicides, new forms of research, has become known as the Green Revolution. There's ongoing debate about the ways and means of this transformation of agriculture, which was based on developing resistant, high-yield seed monotypes and using the azole fungicidal chemicals, which in turn created a dependency on a new agricultural-industrial complex, most of it based in the United States. But there can be no doubt about the science and the way it was organized, from field to laboratory and back again. In what would become the model for organizations such as the Centro Internacional de la Papa, a new Maize and Wheat Improvement Centre was set up in Mexico to monitor rust infestations and research improvements in plant defence. It developed the concept of sentinel fields – fields especially planted as science experiments, to see what is developing that we need to pay attention to, and ensuring we do it quickly and effectively.

The sentinel field concept is the most effective way to do stewardship of the fungal pathogen threat, and they grow all over the world. Small field laboratories are run by field officers who know all the local farmers. Together, they create a first response in the first minutes after a rust outbreak is reported, sometimes standing together on the edge of the field, seed heads in the palms of their hands, rolling them under their fingertips to see if the husk is dry or crumbling. Their microscopes usually confirm what their eyes and hands have already told them. Fungal pathogen stewards are exemplary at remembering that fieldwork means actual fields, so parallel technology is designed to be used where fungi are found. Considering fungal pathogens spread so quickly, it's actually quite hard to grow them in the laboratory, especially rust fungus. To identify a fungus, it must be grown and observed and analysed on the spot, no time to waste, just like the scientists of other eras who knew to press and dry blighted leaves before they went brown and lost their usefulness. Increasingly, inside labs close to the sentinel fields, there are small, cheap, transportable gene sequencers that tell researchers exactly what is going on there, with not quite the detail of main office labs, but enough to be sent off, to become part of the global databases of pathogenic fungi, part of the line around the world. We don't yet have sequencers that plug into smartphones, but they are close.[163] In the meantime, there are apps that can be downloaded to smartphones that enable them to 'sniff' plants and detect sickness in the odours they give off, and the information can be sent to whoever needs it, the university or the agrichemical company, so they can tell which fungicides or seed variants to sell the farmer next time.

In 1998, when a scientist from the International Maize and Wheat Improvement Centre was sent a sample from a sentinel field in Uganda, he saw immediately that it was a new form of wheat rust. He called it strain Ug99 (named because it came from Uganda and the year they confirmed its presence was 1999, just as the presence of COVID-19 was confirmed in 2019) and he sent round the alerts. But, for the next few years, nothing. Ug99 appeared to have gone away on its own. Then, in 2002, it came back, this time appearing in sentinel fields planted all over East Africa, with a hundred different varieties of wheat, almost all of them infected with red, spore-filled sores. Ug99 had turned into a monster from the agronomists' nightmares – a hopeful monster. In a wonderful example of poetry and scientific language intersecting, a 'hopeful monster' is defined as a living organism with a single but profound mutation, which may be enough to establish an entirely new evolutionary lineage within a single bound or leap (its less poetic name is saltational evolution).[164] Not the deft little steps of haplotype change, but huge strides in seven-league genetic boots. Not everyone in gene science is convinced about hopeful monsters, but if they exist at all, we're most likely to see them in fungal evolution, particularly given how varieties like Ug99 learn resistance so quickly.[165]

When gene sequencing was done on samples of the pathogen sent back from the sentinel fields in East Africa, the scientists found that it hadn't started out there, but came originally from the wheat-growing areas around the Himalayas, where two rust types combined (one of which was known to be quite inclined to combine with any-thing blown its way) to make something new. There had been rust pathogens that had come from this area before, but nothing quite like Ug99. And it's now been found in Asia, Europe, America and Australia.[166] Ug99 becomes more virulent and resistant every time it leaps, with increased aggressiveness and a tolerance of high tem-peratures. One of its new strains is actually called the *Warrior* strain, and another *Triticale aggressive*. That's scientists using every means at their disposal to flag up a sentinel event. Or, to put it another way, wheat rust in the form of Ug99 is potentially the *Acinetobacter baumannii* of the pathogenic fungal world. It was so bad, Norman Borlaug himself came to inspect his old enemy, even though he was ill and less mobile than he had been, but he still needed to see the devastated Kenyan fields with his own eyes and to check that his part of the line was holding under the strain. Then he went back to the HQ of the International Maize and Wheat Improvement Centre (still in Mexico, where he founded it) and secured the grants and commitment needed to fight back.

By 2009, the outbreak in East Africa had been contained, using the systematic approach that has been working for half a century. New fungicides were formulated for use on the fields, and updated advice was given about spotting the fungus should it reoccur. Funding for the labs and sentinel fields was reassessed and increased. Farmers replanted their fields with new forms of seed, bred from wheat with natural high resistance to Ug99. So far, they are holding a good, clean, rust-free line. It was time for a change, anyway – good agricultural stewardship says wheat varieties should be replaced every ten to fifteen years, if blight is to be managed. Just like their colleagues in the antibacterial world, scientists are working on genetic solutions to the pathogen, so they can dial down its virulence. They've identified the components that control resistance learning in Ug99 and its variants, and they are working towards being able to switch some or all of them off. We're not there yet, just as we're not quite there with *Acinetobacter Baumannii*, but we have a good plan.

In other labs, scientists work on gene transfer – splicing out likely useful genes and incorporating them into plant cells. This has nothing to do with selective breeding (no plant sex, no parents). DNA allows us to identify markers of use, and genetic modification allows them to be added from one plant to another. Depending on your point of view, GM crops are either saviours or monsters. But, in reality, they are neither. They are part of the response, no guarantees. They need herbicides to be used alongside them, as adjuncts, so no miracles. And, well, fungi are smart. Sometimes, I hear echoes of the dreams of a new Eden used by advocates for GM techniques, but they should be more careful. GM works well in the lab, delivers clearly quantifiable results and thus is readily adaptable to the academic journal article, but it gets fewer gold stars in the field. Genetic modification is good at increasing yields, but less good at developing resistance to fungi or viruses. It should get better as we get better at dealing with individual genes. But we're not there yet either.[167]

If you ask the Centro Internacional de la Papa, they'll tell you that talking about GM is a bit, well, *pasado*. What they would like is what the antibacterial stewards are starting to get – the ability to use big-data analytical techniques on their gene banks and catalogues. They'd like to be able to use artificial intelligence (AI) to work through the digital details that it takes humans decades to work through, which are especially complicated in the potato genome. They'd like AI to find and suggest new genetic combinations to defeat fungal pathogens and all the other enemies of the potato, so that they can get on with the work of making even better, stronger, more nutri-dense varieties and send them out into the world. And, for the CIP, big data is only truly big when it incorporates learning from the Guardians of the Potato, high up in their fields in the Andes. The potato AI revolution is coming, and it will be participatory. It's done its learning in advance. Farmers, social scientists, anthropologists and field agronomists will all be part of the process that guides the terms of the machine learning, as well as the AI programming specialists and geneticists. Potatoes set the pace.

Other sentinel events have come and gone. In 1973, wheat rust in Australia caused billions of Australian dollars' worth of damage, in today's money. Coffee rust wiped out 40 per cent of Colombia's production between 2008 and 2011. Enjoy bananas while they last. When you eat a banana, the small faint marks in the fruit's centre are shadows of the seeds bananas used to make when they were in their wild forms, in New Guinea, where they first grew. Farmers cultivated them in the orchards and gardens near their villages, and because they wanted maximum fruit, minimum seeds, they selected forms that eventually became seedless and sterile, so the only way to reproduce them was to propagate cuttings from their rhizome root systems. So, no banana families, just banana clones. The first superstar cultivated banana form was Gros Michel, and the reason we no longer recognize it is because it was wiped out by the 1970s. One Gros Michel banana plant caught a fungal disease, and then spread it to all the other identical plants in the banana plantation. And, from there, around the world. *Fusarium* wilt – more easily remembered as Panama disease – enters the banana plant through its root system and then spreads through the vascular system of the plant, eating stems, poisoning leaves, eventually killing the entire entity. Panama disease is the kind of fungal pathogen that has very thick cell walls, not easily breached, resilient. It has what are known as 'resting spores'. Banana scientists call this ability 'notorious' (this is language being used as sentinel, like describing *Acinetobacter baumannii*'s abilities as 'uncanny'). Panama disease fungi lie around in the soil, resting. Good long rests – for decades (possibly as long as thirty years). Whole generations of farmers can come and go, and they forget the bananas that grew in their fields once died, so they plant more of them, and they die again, and livelihoods and lives are utterly ruined.

We have found a new form of banana, called Cavendish. We thought it could resist Panama disease, but we know better now. Cavendish is a global banana monoculture, cloned, sterile. Panama disease has taken on a slightly different form, one that likes Cavendish just as much as humans, and it eats the whole plant. I can't put it more clearly than one of the world's leading plant pathologists, who works in Florida (which, along with Hawaii, is one of the US's two main banana-growing regions): 'Few options exist for managing this lethal disease.'[168] Panama disease is hard to recognize until it's too late, and so it's difficult to treat with chemicals, either distributed via the roots or injected into the stems of the plant. We've tried to treat the soil with chemicals and heat to destroy the spores while they rest, but neither approach works entirely, and there are always one or two left behind, and it only ever takes one or two, and in the meantime the heat or the chemicals are hugely damaging to the rest of the soil. Digging in other soils that suppress spores (they don't seem to like clay and certain minerals) is a limited option. Digging out infected plants has to be done with great precision, at exactly the right time of year (after the rains), and the field tools used have to be completely sterilized. Farmers of smallholdings, where bananas or banana family plants are a staple crop, often share tools.[169] For them, the advice is wrangled down to simplicity: dig out infected plants and sterilize all tools thoroughly, not with a chemical that has to be paid for, but with fire.

193

There are labs that are looking for allies for our crops from elsewhere in the microbiological universe: fungi and bacteria that eat fungal pathogens. It's a strategy that might work, but it's, well, preclinical – a long way off – and in the meantime, the Cavendish banana may disappear completely. Ultimately, we'll probably have to go back to the jungles of New Guinea and seek out an original wild form, with seeds, that is able to resist wilt and breed on its own, as nature intended. We've found a few of these, but they don't taste the way we expect a banana to taste, and they look funny because they have more seeds, so they won't be any use in a smoothie. Plus, their yield is poor, so no one can make a living from farming them (or shipping them, or distributing them). All that may be left to us is the strange synthetic banana flavour used in cheap confectionery, because the Panama disease fungi will have eaten everything else. This is almost certainly the answer to the question, 'Who will eat the last banana on Earth, and how will they feel?' It will be Panama disease fungi, and they will feel nothing but satisfied and sleepy.

All those different kingdoms of pathogenic microbes, bacteria and fungi are floating around our atmosphere, and we are growing less able to deal with them. Our world is becoming, to borrow from the work of the leading expert in coffee rust, 'a grudging and fragile accommodation' with species – with universes – we cannot see. So an important step forward in combatting fungal pathogens is our less muddled understanding that there is no Eden waiting for us,

no overall victory waiting to be won. Perfect resistance and suffi-
ciency of yield isn't going to be possible. So now we are playing
for the draw, for sustainable intensity (or intensive sustainability),
for the agricultural equivalent of the long second age of antibiotics
that we hope our stewards and scientists are negotiating for us in
another part of the university, holding a line that is a draw and also
an accommodation. Whatever it is, it holds back Horsemen. Against
Pestilence and Famine there is one shared, equivalent goal: to tackle
antimicrobial resistance wherever we find it.

It might be time for a couple of new acronyms that cohere under
the antimicrobial resistance (AMR) banner: ABR, for antibacterial
resistance, and AFR, for antifungal resistance. This isn't just about
different disciplines working together. There is a very direct threat
from the fungal world to animals and humans. Out of the 8,000
fungal species which are pathogenic or parasitical, 625 of them
have developed a taste for vertebrates (anything with a spine).
Amphibians are our sentinel species for fungi that kill animals.
Fungi like amphibians because they are cold-blooded, and because
they can eat them through their skin, outside in. Amphibians
facilitate fungi travel, continent by continent, because of the trade
in rare species. When people collect rare salamanders, they also
collect their skin fungi. 'Thanks for the ride,' the fungi say when
they get to a new terrarium, and they hop off and find another
reptile to colonize and adapt to and feed on. Fungal pathogens
are wiping out amphibian species at a faster rate than any other
kind of living creature on our planet. At first, the acceleration of
amphibian extinction was 'only recognized as a global phenom-

enon' (science's way of saying, 'This is a thing'). Now we know it's fungal pathogens doing the wiping out, and we're working to combat it, using everything from genetics to biosecurity to habitat preservation and amphibian arks (in which select species that would otherwise go extinct will be maintained in captivity until they can be secured in the wild).[170] All of it is stewardship. But it's too late for many species, including the beautiful black and yellow species of fire salamander native to the Netherlands, the last of which disappeared in 2010.[171]

Being a species with a fairly decent existing immune response to threats like viruses and bacteria doesn't help when it comes to fungi. Take bats, with their highly mobile metabolisms and agile inflammatory mechanisms. In the north-eastern United States, in 2006, entire colonies of several different species of bat were found to have died during their hibernation in caves. Each bat had a dusting of white powder on its muzzle, ears and wings, as if its last meal had been coated in icing sugar. Because no one knew what it was, ninety-seven post-mortems were done on tiny bat corpses. The powder was found to be a fungus, which had infected its host by penetrating its skin, sending hyphae tendrils into tissue, through hair follicles and sweat glands. Outside in, just like with the amphibians. None of the bats had any of their hibernation fat stores left – all of it, and them, eaten to death by a fungal pathogen (provisionally called bat white-nose syndrome) no one knew anything about at all before 2006: not where it had come from, nor whether it travelled on the wind where its victims flew or whether it was just resting somewhere in a chilly cave, waiting.[172]

Next stop, us. Three hundred species of pathogenic fungi seem to have acquired a specific taste for humans, beyond just being part of our microbiological universe. Humans get and keep most of their fungal pathogens on their skin, because healthy human body temperatures don't suit them. Temperature is one of the ways we've been living with fungal pathogens as part of our own evolutionary process and mostly our immune systems can manage them.[173] But some fungal pathogens are quite happy at more than thirty-seven degrees Celsius, the temperature of a compromised immune system. They are opportunistic, hanging around hospital critical care wards, looking for people already ill with cancer, with HIV, with cystic fibrosis in their lungs, complicated and thickened by biofilms of bacterial infection. They are looking for people with strong allergic reactions, or with nasty, hospital-admittance-requiring cases of flu and other viruses, especially in people with underlying health conditions.[174] And they are hoping to hop a ride on any of the medical devices that pierce the skin or are carefully inserted to support breathing, but either way provide an easy route past epidermal defensive mechanisms, deep into the fungi-friendly tissue in the interior of human bodies. In 2015, a significant outbreak was caused by one single infected ear thermometer and a strain of fungal pathogen that simply ignored the careful disinfectant procedures used between each patient (remember, warm weather and travel, a few of their favourite things – even if it's a warm body and the journey isn't always intercontinental). Whenever antibiotic stewards talk about the risks of bacterial infection in the acute setting, they are also (even when they don't realize it) talking about fungal pathogens. *Acinetobacter baumannii*, meet *Aspergillus fumigatus*. Welcome to the handrail.[175]

Aspergillus fumigatus is a fungal pathogen with the kind of power and range that *Acinetobacter baumannii* can only dream of. It is found across the kingdoms and continents of all living things, infecting whatever it finds there, from wheat (where we treat it by spraying the fields with azole-class fungicides), to penguins, to people. Professor Matt Fisher, who works on fungal pathogen epidemiology at Imperial College, not far away from Esmita and her colleagues, is my steward of choice for this section, and his research career, like Sarah Gurr's, underpins and symbolizes the direction of fungal pathogen research in our time. At the University of California, at Berkeley, Matt was part of a team investigating valley fever, which affects humans with something like flu and is inflicted by a fungal pathogen that lives mostly in the soil of the south-western United States and parts of Central America. When the report on amphibian extinctions was published, everyone in the field pitched in with the research effort to hold this new part of the line on behalf of creatures all too easily lost. Today, Matt continues to investigate the emergence of new fungal pathogens that we don't know about (like the ones in the bat cave), and also the emergence of new dangerous forms of fungal pathogens we are already well aware of. Part of his stewardship is the maintenance of Imperial's library of 600 separate isolates of genome-sequenced *Aspergillus fumigatus* microbes – the biggest in the world. He's explained to me how *Aspergillus* lives all around us, like radon or UV light – a background hazard, until suddenly it's not. Matt calls these points, where *Aspergillus* suddenly remembers to compete aggressively, 'hot spots' – although they may not be hot, just really active, like Wi-Fi.

We are increasingly finding *Aspergillus* hot spots where we least expect them. There is more *Aspergillus fumigatus* in cities than there is in the countryside. It's evolved with deft little steps to become more deadly than wild-type infections, and it's found in the very worst place imaginable: horticultural flower beds in close proximity to city-centre hospitals.[176] Flower beds are supposed to be good for patients looking out of ward windows. Hospitals increasingly have space for their own gardens as alternative sites of recovery, which are generally thought to be better for everyone than looking out over barren concrete car parks or stone and glass atria. Flower beds have been planted with bulbs that are supposed to be pretreated with azoles, but which are increasingly resistant. Spores of the fungus that grows on them blow up and around in the air, on to visitors to the hospital, through the ward windows, on to handrails, hanging around, meeting other microbes, before finally heading down into the lungs of people who don't have the immune systems to cope with them. It has a medical name now, as well as its fungi plant taxonomy: aspergillosis. Aspergillosis, along with other fungal pathogens that have developed a taste for humans, is estimated to kill more than a million of us each year, worldwide.

We treat aspergillosis in intensive care in the same way we treat it in intensive farming. We use azole-class fungicides, with modified delivery mechanisms. There are only four classes of azoles, and *Aspergillus fumigatus* is resistant to nearly all of them, in whatever settings they are used. It doesn't even have to learn quickly – with processes like flower-bulb-to-people transfer, resistant fungal path-ogens are already there, embedded in the tissue of a vulnerable patient, doing their damage. When azole fungicides stop working in fields, farmers and agrochemical companies tweak the formulation to try to stay one step ahead of the outbreak. Something similar is happening in hospitals. We're trying to make the formulations we have work better, by ensuring they are properly targeted, so the azole goes where it is supposed to, and not anywhere else. It's the same sort of thinking that happens with antibiotics to lengthen the second age. Narrow their spectrum, make them work only where they are most needed, so they are prevented from wandering off and learning resistance along the way.

There is a new kind of delivery mechanism which gives added precision to the process of targeting aspergillosis: azole compounds delivered by inhaler, drawn deep into the lungs where the fungi lurk, hitting them there, not waiting for medication to make its slow systemic way round the body.[177] We're well on the way from preclinical to clinical applications, which is good because, apart from azoles, there are very few other kinds of antifungal drugs that can be used on the humans who need them. Where they are used, it must be with great care and as a last resort. Non-azole antifungal treatments are very strong. They may well poison the fungal pathogen, but they can also end up poisoning the patient. Intensive care is a tough place to hold the line.[178] Antifungal stewardship requires knowledge of the isolate library, the field, the flower bed, the hospital ward and the patient, all as part of the same process, all at the same time.

Where antibiotic stewards go, antifungal stewards can readily follow. And not just by working together, but, increasingly by being the same person, a real full-spectrum antimicrobial steward: a pharmacist. The pharmacist on the ward round can monitor fungal pathogen and bacterial infection. They can make sure the lab tests that come back tell the full microbiological story of their patient, and remind everyone that it may not be the antibiotics that are failing, but the antifungals. They can help radiologists spot fungal spores on their CT scans or chest X-rays. They can make sure that prescription and delivery of antifungals is appropriate, and adjust or de-escalate where they, as steward, see fit. They know about drug interactions. They can keep an eye on source control – all those catheters and tubes and microbes and ear thermometers on the surfaces of which fungi hope to cadge a free ride. They'll do their best to report back their findings, but the surveillance system for fungal pathogen resistance in people is not yet as good as the ones for bacterial resistance. The smart-surface work being done to combat antibiotic resistance has applications in antifungal resistance: copper alloys used in hospital water pipes could also be used in air-conditioning systems, because otherwise fungal pathogens thrive in their inner pipes and water tanks.[179] In the meantime, no need to guess about the still little understood world of fungal pathogens in the hospital. Ask the pharmacist. There should be one on the ward round.[180]

To understand the true scope of antifungal stewardship, we should step back from horrified contemplation of what we used to think were harmless, brightly coloured hospital flower beds doing their best to cheer us up, and broaden our gaze out to Canada, where today there are ten million hectares of land producing wheat, in the largest fields ever cultivated in the history of our world. It is two Canadian wheat cultivars that provided the new Ug99-resistant strains for the world's new wheat seed stocks. The cultivars have names, because it's easier to remember than long numbers. So, up against *Warrior* and *Triticale aggressive* rust fungus are *Peace* and *AC Cadillac*. So far, *Peace* and *AC Cadillac* are winning (annoying for the rider of the red horse, as well as the black). And, unsurprisingly, Canada is a world leader in generating antifungal research strategy. The Canadian Institute for Advanced Research (CIFAR) is one of the first multidiscipli-nary organizations to focus on the 'exciting opportunity' of fungal pathogen research. Sarah and Matt are two of the fellows in their programme, Fungal Kingdom: Threats & Opportunities. CIFAR's team has written the equivalent of the *Mosul Trauma Report* for fungal pathogens: *One Health: Fungal Pathogens of Humans, Animals and Plants*. Not only does it explain the complexities of the cross-kingdom effects of fungal pathogens, it also reminds us that there is a very special place in the line for people who write really great reports as well as being capable of doing epic science. The work is clear and fascinating, terrifying and readily quotable: 'The fungal kingdom is generally neglected when it comes to considering catastrophic risks to humanity.'

The report also says that fungi are 'exquisitely responsive to environmental perturbation, which can exacerbate their deleterious effects', as we can see in the case of a fungus that destroys soy bean crops, which has learned to travel in hurricane season. In the last half century, it has skipped from Hawaii to South America, and, in September 2004, came as the first soy bean pathogen ever recorded in

North America courtesy of a very bumpy ride on Hurricane Ivan.[181] More hurricanes occur because of disrupted weather patterns, so more fungi will be carried along with them, probably. Although, if we think back to the steamships crossing the oceans, before we got going on the climate, we should also remember that it doesn't have to be climate-change-induced freak weather events that move fungi around. Some of the most threatening fungi of all don't care what happens to temperatures – up or down, it's all the same to them. It could be ordinary wind, nothing special, just seasonal, blowing exactly when we expect it to, where it has always blown for as long as our landmasses have looked this way, our rivers deep and mountains high. Just wind is all it takes. Biotroph fungal spores (like those of wheat rust) in particular like to be aerially dispersed, and can survive for weeks on wind alone. Meteorologists track and quantify fungi's airborne dispersal routes, which means machine learning and high-performance computational resources to combine global weather data, atmospheric physics, wind and temperature patterns, trajectory model data and network analysis. Combining this with our understanding of specific fungi varieties, down to their genetic underthings, together with sentinel and agricultural field stations, we can create a huge map of the winds of the Earth, where they blow, when, and what they carry.[182]

Which brings us back to Ug99. We're very certain that it originated in the near-Himalayas, because the genetics backs up the meteorology. To get to the sentinel fields where the distinct resistance patterns were first observed and calculated, the pathogen would have ridden winds that blew from Nepal, across the Middle East into

Africa. From there, a direct route leads into the huge wheat-growing archipelago that stretches from Ethiopia, Uganda and Kenya to the eastern and southern countries of Africa (Tanzania, Malawi, Mozambique, Zambia and Zimbabwe). Across the archipelago, scientists have found that there are nodes of high connectivity where fungal spores are spread faster and more efficiently by prevailing winds, turning endemic spore activity (the small outbreak of Ug99 in 1999) into multiple outbreaks (from 2002 onwards) or even epidemics. Nowhere is a more effective node of connectivity than the African Rift Valley, the depth and length of which channels winds both north to south and south to north – epidemiologists in plant science call it the flyway of fungal spores.

Between October and December, the spores ride the winds that blow south along the valley. As they encounter plant material that they like to eat, they do, developing resistance to the features that make it less palatable. In Kenya, most wheat grown is durum wheat. Long thought to be more resistant to wheat rust than other varieties, it isn't anymore, because, from 2002, Ug99 blew over it, and got a taste for it, and spread what it had learned. Between June and August, the winds and the spores head back north along the valley, and on beyond the African continent. The point at which winds from Africa head into the Arabian peninsula, and from there to central Europe, Asia and beyond (and back again), is Yemen, the last of the islands in the wheat archipelago, and it acts as a green bridge between Europe, Africa and eventually Asia. The country has two main climate zones – the eastern, mostly desert equivalent, and the western, which looks more like Sudan or Ethiopia than Arabia, with higher rainfall.

Winds strengthen as they blow through Yemen, concentrating their spore density, depositing and picking up new resistance forms from crops in the country. Yemen is, all at the same time, a spore donor country, a high point of spore transfer and a zone of intercontinental spore transfer.[183]

Yemen has been at war within and beyond its own borders since 2015. But despite almost everything else falling apart, somehow agriculture is trundling on, with more wheat being planted than before war broke out. In 2016, Yemeni agriculturalists picked up a ferocious strain of Ug99 in their fields.[184] But war means Yemen can't take advantage of the gains made against Ug99 from the East African outbreaks, because there is no peace, and also no *Peace* or *AC Cadillac* wheat cultivar seed stock. Communications are bad, infrastructure is all but smashed to pieces, and the chemicals that are needed as fungicides can't be distributed together with the guidance on usage and agricultural stewardship. The relevant experts aren't able to move around the country, and the sentinel fields with their labs and personnel that would test the ever-evolving strains that blow across the land of the green bridge no longer exist. They were lucky to identify their strain of Ug99 at all.

Yemen is still farming now, but cut off from the rest of the world. If Ug99 is still there, feeding and learning, it hasn't been tracked or monitored. Most global organizations have withdrawn their staff from the country because it's simply too dangerous to work there, and they watch as best they can from beyond its borders. They've lost most of their home-grown agricultural scientists in Yemen, so there's no almost no agricultural science being done there. Any sentinel fields are now gone, and there is no one to watch and warn the rest of the world when the wind blows north and east, and the spores head off across the Middle East and then to Iran. Iran has had dry weather in the last few years, so any fungal pathogen progress will have been slowed, but we know they can learn drought resilience, so it's thought to be only a question of time before something like Ug99 gets to the huge wheat farms that provide for the giant bread-basket of Pakistan and India.[185] When the wind blows south through Yemen, it will carry spores back down the Rift Valley, hopping across the wheat archipelago. At the other end of the African Rift Valley channel, it gets to southern Africa, where there is some (not much, but enough) inter-regional air transfer between there and Oceania. Air that blows off central South Africa arrives on the coastal waters of Australia in fifteen days, and Ug99 may be able to survive that long in one of its new varieties. It won't take much, just a few spores of a hopeful monster, touching down, spreading out.[186] Ninety per cent of the world's wheat is vulnerable to Ug99, and the more it spreads, the fewer varieties there will be to breed resistance from, to replace stocks. We may have normal transmission mechanisms, predicted resistance agility, the best mathematical meteorological modelling money can buy, but the blood-red horse of War keeps clip-clopping up behind Famine, a reminder that their best work is always done together.

The rider of the red horse has a particular interest in fungal path-ogens and doing what he can to help them realize their dreams of travel. Twenty-five miles from the centre of Rome, and providing one of the last green lungs of the city, is the forest of Castelporziano. Roman emperors had villas in the forest (the president of Italy uses one there still, as a country residence), and the flora and fauna look similar today as they did in imperial times. It has oaks and brushwood and poplars and ash trees. Above all, literally and symbolically, there are stone pines – some of which are centuries old, and officially designated as arboreal monuments – planted for their pine nuts and their ability to anchor otherwise sandy soils. There's a fungal pathogen – *Hetrobasidion annosum* – which attacks the roots of stone pines. In Europe, it isn't a problem. Stone pines and fungus live together, not productively, but not dangerously, neither side seeking the win, content to live with the draw. Not so with the version of the fungus that comes from North America, which has the smallest amount of different genetic material, making it fatal to stone pines.

At the end of the twentieth century, the stone pines of Castelporziano did something they very rarely did. They died, quite suddenly and mysteriously. Not all of them, but enough for their human caretakers to notice that something odd was going on. In 2004, Italian mycologists were able to extract the DNA of the fungus that had killed them. Initially, it looked like *Hetrobasidion annosum*, but not when they looked again and sequenced their findings. In it, they found haplotypes from North American DNA – eastern North American DNA, to be precise (which they could be) – that had become incorporated with the Italian version, settling in effectively and starting to compete aggressively. *Hetrobasidion annosum* doesn't spread on the wind, it can't survive being airborne; it likes to travel commercially and it can survive in cut hewn wood for long periods, so it was most likely the fungus had been directly imported from America, in some of its wood products.

But the forest of Castelporziano has never been open to the public; it's a nature reserve. Admission is for emperors and presidents only. Except for a few weeks in the Second World War, when regiments of the US Fifth Army occupied the estate and buildings as part of their push through Italy into the rest of Europe to defeat fascism. They drove their jeeps along roads they cut, marking them off with wooden fence posts. Lorries trundled in and out all day and all night, loading and unloading supplies on wooden pallets and in crates, all known to be made of untreated cuts of US stone pine. Lots and lots of wood from America. And the fungus spread from the timber on the ground, through the soil, into the root systems of the Italian natives, slowly – fungi timescales often are, especially those that live in trees – so it was decades before the disease symptoms became visible, but by then it was too late for some of the stone pines of Castelporziano. The identification of the specific forms of fungus enables the disease to be managed, so the stone pines should be protected in future.

Military operations can have long-term effects on natural ecosystems. Just a nod from a couple of passing Horsemen, and trees that bore witness to the rise and fall of the Roman Empire were defeated by an untreated fence post and a fungus that was prepared to take its time.[187]

It was a different, contingent chain of events that brought *Phytoph-thora infestans* to Ireland in 1845. The Great Famine of the nineteenth century was brutal from the outset, a misunderstood natural disaster made catastrophic by British inaction and a brutal, cruel lack of concern from those in authority. Famine in the twentieth century, on the other hand, came from drought bearing down on subsistence farming (and gave us the images we always associate with the effects of the rider of the black horse today). So far, famine in the twenty-first century has never been accidental, or inevitable. It is always man-made, war-made. The Great Famine of our time is happening in war-torn Yemen, both forms of devastation in one poor, benighted place. Famine in Yemen is one of the agents of a very modern civil war. The country is split into two factions, both supported by for-eign powers, and much of the violence inflicted is by rockets and missiles, from afar. There is not much ground engagement, except for asymmetric incursions and bouts of sudden terroristic violence from small brutal groups to quell and terrify the locals. Yemen was always poor, reliant for most of its food on imports – coastline being the only thing it isn't short of – with two big ports (Aden and Hudaydah) bringing in food, medicines and most of the fuel that the population needs to survive, all of which were stored in huge warehouse facilities and distributed via a decent road and bridge network across the country. Only the amount of coastline remains unchanged today. The ports can import food when one side says they can and lifts its blockade.

When the warehouses are unloaded and the lorries drive away, they are stopped at the other side's blockades of bridges and roads, and the food and supplies they carry are diverted or sold, although as the years have passed and war continues in the ascendant, there are fewer bridges and roads that remain intact enough to blockade. There have been cholera outbreaks on a medieval scale (so Pestilence joins the group). There is no healthcare system left to speak of. Yemen is officially the world's worst humanitarian disaster, and there has been no failure of the rains, no Ug99, no exceptional heat or cold, no grinding of the tectonic plates beneath its landscape or off its coastline. Every element of the crisis is entirely man-made.

Nor is Yemen's man-/war-made famine something new. Famine is not a feature particular to modern asymmetric war or low-intensity conflict or transnational or hybrid wars, or whatever academics in political science departments are calling them now. Famine has always been with us, in the much older forms of warfare that are still being waged in our world, those forms that are comfortably familiar to the Horsemen, not just on the liberation battlefields of Mosul, but in sieges everywhere. Sieges constitute the most drastic and direct confrontation between civilians and the military.

Sieges are military blockades of cities and towns with the intention of achieving defeat by attrition of supplies.[188] Starvation is a military tactic, although the modern variant prevents not only supplies getting through, but also humanitarian aid, from recognizably humanitarian agencies (and it's all in violation of UN Resolution 2417, which states that using starvation of civilians as a method of warfare may constitute a war crime).[189] The sieges the Horsemen knew from Dürer's time lasted months, even years, until cities were ground down to almost nothing, and the besiegers could eventually rampage through them and take what little remained. Sieges are much shorter now. Towns are rarely completely cut off for more than a few weeks (and with social media, just like at Mosul, none are ever completely cut off, so although we may not be able to get to them, we can follow along with what's happening in real time).

But the effects are very much the same. Supplies run short, black markets establish themselves, looting and theft aggravate and concentrate existing hatreds among those besieged, and malnutrition and disease spread across the battered streets and into every home. In Syria, where there were twenty-four separate sieges of varying intensity, imposed by all sides in the fighting, from 2011 to 2018, two and a half million people were affected, pinned back into ruined buildings, all egress denied to them, constantly pounded towards submission. Key infrastructure was targeted first – schools, hospitals, municipal buildings, utility complexes – then whatever or whoever was left standing.[190] The Horsemen know from experience that the longer a place holds out, the worse its fate will be. These sieges ended with surrender for those who survived, population displacement and (usually) scorched earth at water sources, agricultural smallholdings and the remaining food stores. And then starvation – and the science of starvation never changes, whatever the time or place.

Siege economics never change, either. It is not that there is nothing. For nothing, you need weather-induced famine, wiping out all living things as far as their failing eyes can see – nothing on the bone-dry horizon. But man-made famine means hunger, not absence of food. There is always food somewhere, and medicines, and supplies, sitting in warehouses or occupier-friendly distribution points, or on the black market.

But all of it – as well as the fuel needed to move vehicles and the water needed to drink and cook, and power to turn on stoves more than once a day (refrigeration is usually a long-forgotten dream) – is shockingly, prohibitively expensive. In such times, no one has jobs or money worth the mention, so they can't afford even the most basic foodstuffs, and they become dependent on foreign aid (which is usually stuck in the ports, or at the checkpoints, awaiting un-blockading). Perhaps the Horseman who brings famine recognizes that this is the essence of his work, because he has always carried a pair of balances in his hand, never equally or fairly weighted. On one side, a burdensome amount of money, to buy what is on the other side – not enough, poor-quality food. And wherever it happens in the world, and for whatever reason, the highest costs are paid by children. Paid and hardly ever refunded, worst of all when the price is set in wartime. Bridges and tunnels, road networks and cities are relatively easily rebuilt. Children, not so much.

The construction of our skeletons starts before we are born, when our cells split into all kinds of person-making material and begin to build. At this stage, it's as if scaffolding is going up. And not just in our hard tissues (although that's the easiest to imagine) – the same process is going on in our soft tissues, particularly in our brains, but also our kidneys, livers, hearts, everything. We do a lot of our growing, proportionately, before we are born and during the first thousand days after our birth day, especially our long bones (in our arms and legs), which grow quickly compared to the relatively slow development of our trunk, the axis of our physical being. We should – we must – live off good-quality breast milk for six months, but after that we need more nutritional food alongside. Then we need good regular feeding in time for our second growth spurt, in adolescence. After that, we reach maturity, when the scaffolding comes down. We won't get any taller, and our bone growth slows. There are a few variations for gender and age, but it's how all human beings are built from scratch, our blueprint, and all the processes are preprogrammed into our cells, dependent on signals from around our body, no matter where or when we live on earth.

This preprogrammed process is disrupted by malnutrition, when good regular feeding of nutritious food becomes something less. Malnutrition occurs when the food available to human beings is not only of insufficient quantity, but is also insufficiently nourishing. Starvation and malnutrition aren't necessarily the same thing. If humans are briefly starved, then its effects are transient. If they are malnourished for long periods of time, the effects become permanent. And the very worst time for this to happen is during the first thousand days of a human's life, when the scaffolding is going up. Malnutrition isn't just the extreme forms we can recognize on the news, like the famines we saw in the twentieth century – that's severe acute malnutrition (SAM, for short). We need to stop only seeing SAM when we think of famine, because we now recognize slower forms of famine as being equally dangerous, where it takes much longer to see its effects, but they get there in the end. Undernutrition is malnutrition by other means, in the long run, and every bit as bad for us.

Undernutrition is the most dangerous component of food in-security. It happens when crops fail – because a fungus that had been sleeping for thirty years suddenly woke up and ate a banana crop, or obliterated a wheat field – when there is nothing to eat or sell, and the household economy is challenged, and a family looks into the future and sees empty shelves and nothing but dust and cobwebs in its cooking pots. Food insecurity also happens in sieges and conflict, and anywhere there are refugees. Symptoms of food in-security are things like reducing portion sizes, planning fewer meals per day (one, for instance), cutting spending on food, borrowing food from whoever may have some, spending all day waiting for a humanitarian agency supply truck that may never come. Quantity is prioritized over quality, so the amount on the plate may be the same or more, and it's filling, but it's nutritionally valueless. Or the food available is completely different from what a child is used to eating, so their bodies don't know how to process it, so they don't. Or it's raw, or cold, because fuel is scarce, so pans are heated up once a day and then left to cool slowly, allowing for bacterial contamination. Or it's under-ripe or overripe, old, bad (cheap) or spoiled.

Food-insecure mothers give up food to feed the rest of their family, and stress or displacement may cause them to stop breast-feeding. If they are pregnant, their malnutrition becomes their unborn child's malnutrition.[191] Malnutrition also has indirect effects. A child returned to Mosul was asked for her strongest memory of occupation. Great, terrible sadness, was the reply, at the memory of how her parents struggled every single day to get enough food for her baby sister.

When food doesn't nourish us sufficiently, it's because it's missing macronutrients, the elements of which we mostly understand because they give us the energy we need to live: proteins, fats and carbohydrates. And then there are the micronutrients, which are tiny but powerful – by their presence and their absence. Micronutrients are minuscule amounts of substances that enable our bodies to produce enzymes, hormones and other chemicals that generate the physiological processes that enable our cells to follow the blueprint. They provide the messaging system whereby our cells are told to grow or develop or change or react, preferably at the same time and at the original preprogrammed pace. The most important ones are iron, iodine and vitamin A. If these micronutrients are missing for long enough periods, our body's messaging system begins to be affected. It stops sending out the grow and develop messages, and instead it goes into a kind of survival mode of power conservation.

So, here's what we are looking out for when we want to spot the first visible signs of malnutrition, under-nutrition and micronutrient deficiency in children: growth failure. Or, as it's more depressingly known, wasting and stunting. Stopping construction work is the body's way to adapt to suboptimal growth conditions.[192] When we want to know if a child is malnourished, we could take a blood sample or a hormone panel, but mainly what we do is take out our pair of balances and a (non-elastic) tape, and ask their age. Then we weigh them, and measure how tall they are when standing barefoot, mostly. Upper-body height can also be measured by seating them on a custom-made stool, where distance between the base of the spine and the top of the head is measured. We also measure leg length, and we wrap our tape around their upper arm to see its circumference. Stunting and wasting can happen separately, but mostly they don't. Stunting and wasting frequently coexist, although not necessarily as steady states, so children can move into one phase and out of the other. We are currently settled on the general descriptor that children have multiple measures of anthropometric failure, and that we probably need to work out a better system of metrics, at some point.[193]

There is an international standard of linear growth, which matches age and development and encompasses a full spectrum of heights across populations. And there are lots of variables. Height-for-age standard scores only work for children, not for adolescents, and only if the age of the child is known by their caregiver – and little children aren't reliable at remembering how old they are, if they can talk at all. This is what really big organizations like the WHO are useful for, so let's not forget it. They create and maintain international standards of what children should look like if they eat properly, anywhere in the world, and this is a very good thing for us all to know. If the metrics have to be reworked, then the WHO will implement the changes, across the world. Currently, the WHO Child Growth Standards median defines stunting as impaired growth and development which is two standard deviations below what it should be. Two standard deviations looks like reduced height, low weight, reduced leg length and insufficient skinfold (which is worked out from the pinch test that shows if there is fat under the skin, not just skin, which doesn't spring back into place after we've let go).

What the standard tells us is usually what our eyes have already seen. If the child is thinner than they should be, and shorter than we'd expect, then they are wasted and stunted. For a while, these effects of malnutrition were treated separately, but we know better now, and we know that they are almost always seen together, being more powerful that way, harder to compensate for.[194] We are starting to understand that there is much more that is not visible to the eye or measurable by the balance scale or the tape or the custom-made stool, and this is where the science starts to come in. When it no longer has sufficient access to micronutrients, the body's messaging system restricts itself from putting on weight in fat, or height in bone growth. It's taking the scaffolding down, not everywhere, but from what evolution has calculated to be the less important parts of the construction.

So the skin pinch test is really crucial, beyond the obvious visible reasons. If a child is undernourished, the owner of the body won't have energy to spare to store in fat. Fat is more dynamic than we necessarily realize – doing the pinch test to see how much we have isn't just measuring body shape. Fat is a complex communication system of its own. The presence of fat tells the brain how much energy we have left, and what we can do with it.[195] So without fat, bones don't grow, because fat mass regulates long-bone growth. Leptin, the hormone found in fatty tissue, stimulates bone growth, so shorter leg length may be a good indicator that the body is reducing some growth processes in favour of normal operation in others. The lungs, for instance. Shorter leg length but normal body-trunk growth may indicate that the space being left for the lungs is normal, so that all the energy possible goes into keeping lung function and capacity at an unreduced rate – the means whereby oxygen is moved around our bodies, without which we are dead in minutes.[196] Something similar happens when energy gets spared and diverted to brain development. We call this thrifty growth (scientists call it the thrifty phenotype hypothesis). Activating thrift in development = stunting as survival by other means.

Thrifty growth can only go so far. Stunting and wasting are the forms of malnutrition we can see, which is why it's easier to measure them with a tape and scales. But the really dangerous forms are invisible, and much harder to quantify. The immune function that fights off infectious diseases (bacterial and fungal) is a system, not an organ, and so it doesn't qualify for extra energy. To work properly, the immune system needs micronutrients, just like the rest of the body, from the outset and then on into life. To understand children's immune systems (which is essential, because the system is so fundamental in determining how children will eventually become adults), people need to see beyond the visible, and understand malnutrition as a continuum, an interaction, a process that can't be fixed by food security alone. The line runs strong and solid through the laboratories of the Prendergast Group in London's Queen Mary University, where paediatricians, immunologists, microbiologists and geneticists are exploring the links between infection, immunity and malnutrition. Members of the Group were the first researchers to describe malnutrition as an immunodeficiency syndrome. Syndromes, continuums, co-morbidities – the really important thing they want us all to understand is that malnutrition is more than just 'impaired nutrient assimilation' or 'inadequate food intake'.[197] The Prendergast Group are the stewards of good child nutrition that I know best, and I know them as a collective, because they answer my questions together, some from the meeting room and the rest from video links across the world, from Canada to Zimbabwe, where they conduct their research projects. (One of which is the Health Outcomes, Pathogenesis and Epidemiology of Severe Acute Malnutrition, or HOPE-SAM study – hope, right there, in the name, and of course in the work they do tracking the long-term health of children living with HIV, who are participating in nutritional rehabilitation projects.) Whatever we are talking about comes down to their central focus: malnutrition and immune dysfunction are (their underlining) closely linked. It didn't take much to explain the idea of the Horsemen always riding together to the Prendergast Lab.

They've explained to me just how systematic the immune system is. Immunity is what we call the series of layers that protect us from the outside, microbiological world that would otherwise damage us. The layer we know best is found in our skin, where the outside world meets our inside. There are other areas in our body where this happens (our mouths, or our urinary tracts, for instance) and what they have in common with our skin is the protective epithelial layer, which has its own tiny microbiome chemical universe that reacts quickly to microbes like bacteria or fungi. It blocks them getting any deeper into the body, and it regenerates any cells that have been damaged. It puts up a barrier, stopping infection in its tracks. It fixes what's been broken, as quickly as possible. This layer has a powerful agent to do much of its work: mucus. Mucus is the living creature's very own bespoke biofilm. It has all the power of a bacterial biofilm and even a bit more. It traps microbes, especially bacteria that like to spread by biofilm formation, and stops them joining up or reaching further into the body. Mucus springs into action as soon as it senses invasion. It's busy all day and all night, and we are beginning to understand that in the right quantities, and with the right mucosal chemistry, it has a really significant role to play in antibacterial therapies, and that we should probably be making more of it.[198] Skin, its epithelium and mucus are all thick layers in the immune system, and their correct function assumes health and proper nutrition and hydration. They work best when they aren't scratched or scuffed or wounded, so microbes aren't able to directly access parts of us they really shouldn't get to.

Most of our immune system exists deeper inside our bodies, within the gut barrier layer of the intestine. The intestinal immune system layer is thin (one cell deep), but it can tell the difference between nutrients and water, and toxins and bacteria. It works to keep the good stuff in (so we can use it to grow) and the bad stuff out. It does this in much the same way that the skin's immune layers do, with mucus, and it provides a protective layer for our gut microbiome, which does digestion beyond digestion, so what our intestines can't get through, our very own microbiological universe can. These are layers of immune protection, interacting, learning, holding their lines. But they are not part of the thrifty-growth survival strategy, where the priorities are bones and brain. The intestinal layer only works if it receives enough energy to function. If it doesn't, its barrier effects start to fail. Then, the wrong components can leach into the microbiome and even more directly into the vascular system, where they'll be transported around the body via the blood. Toxins – bad food, environmental contaminants – all affect the microbiome directly, upsetting its balance, impairing its ability to find any nutrients at all, poisoning it, dismantling the shields against infection that evolution has so carefully built for us, undermining our inherent immunity. These are the non-visible effects of malnutrition. One way, beyond weights and measures, to see if this process is happening would be to test the tears of a child. There are antibodies (the agents of the immune system) in tears, or at least there should be, but it may be difficult to systematize tears as biomarkers, because if children are all cried out, it's probably too late anyway.[199]

The scientists of the Prendergast Lab understand the real devil in the detail of malnutrition and immune dysfunction. Malnutrition breaks down our immune systems, so we get infections. Infections reduce our appetite, so we get even more malnourished, and at some point, it doesn't matter if there is enough room for lungs to grow normally, because too much energy is going on fighting infections. All the energy and messages that should be going on putting the scaffolding back up, building the child, are instead spent on fighting infection using diminished means. And when these much-reduced functions try to respond to infections, they stay alerted for much longer than they should, draining chemicals and blood supply that should be trying to get back to normal.[200] Non-normal inflammation responses = chronic inflammation, the kind we see that is the difference between life and death in Ebola cases. Malnutrition causes immune dysfunction, and part of that is chronic inflammation – another reason the scaffolding stays down. No wonder scientists also say that malnourished children have 'a suite of overlapping comorbidities that are poorly understood'.[201] This is what immune dysfunction looks like at its most brutal, and it is both cause and consequence of malnutrition. Round and round it goes. Not enough to eat, not enough nutrition from food when it is available. Frequent exposure to toxins, increasingly short periods between infections. Diminishing immune protection. All against a background of external, environmental suboptimal growth conditions – the best kind of background for Famine to catch up with the rest of the Horsemen and compare notes.

No one is preprogrammed to be malnourished, not even if their ancestors have been farming potatoes in the high thin air of the Andes for thousands of years.[202] Potatoes may be able to adapt to changing nutritional circumstances, but people can't. In 2020, the Centro Internacional de la Papa used its connections with Andean potato farmers and found that almost half of their children were undernourished, mainly through deficiencies in iron and zinc, even though some varieties of potato can give as much as half a day's requirement of these and other nutrients, like vitamin C and B, in their raw or cooked form.[203] And this despite successful campaigns to reduce stunting and the effects of malnutrition in what were mostly lowland and urban areas of Peru. Living in the mountains remains a suboptimal growth environment for children. Their access to healthcare is limited, so, if they get ill – with, say, a chest infection – they are likely to go untreated.[204] And they are very likely to get chest infections, because the highlands are a low-oxygen environment, which is especially bad for children. Hypoxia reduces energy production, which reduces growth and development of the immune system (and we also see it in the children of Tibet and Nepal). And it's frequently cold in the mountains, and if children can't adjust their bodies to the temperature, they'll shiver a lot, which takes up energy that can't be spared. Hoofbeats in the distance, if someone is listening carefully enough, the black horse malingering.

The CIP is listening. And learning that stewardship requires them to have a wider remit than they originally envisioned, beyond all the different kinds of tuber and root-system species they currently look after. They need to be the guardians of the Guardians of the Potato. The CIP is responding by going back to the gene bank to look for varieties with even more nutrients, and distributing potato seed to the farmers with families most at risk of malnutrition. They support a programme that recommends growing and eating other vegetables, and possibly keeping some small animals (guinea pigs and chickens), to increase non-potato-derived nutrition and income sources. And although this is all quite new for them, they are doing some hard thinking about hard mountain lives, about how much work should be done by the smallest family members, and when there should be time for rest and play. They are finding pathways up the mountain to secure not only the next generation of potatoes, but also the next generation of potato farmers, who need to be strong enough to hold the line and do the work the world needs them to do.

Most of the malnourished children in the world live in quite another kind of suboptimal environment: conflict zones, or places that until very recently were conflict zones, or that could be conflict zones again at the drop of the wrong hat. Conflict zones, wherever they are in the world, have one thing in common: explosive weapons. Actually, they have two things in common: explosive weapons and undernourished children. They encounter each other all the time, during the fighting of actual conflicts, or in post-conflict zones, where children finally venture out from the safety of their dark basements and go to play, to school, to work, and along the way pick up or tread on things they shouldn't, and the filthy, germ-ridden soil of the war-torn nation is blown deep past all the protective immune-system layers, directly into their blood and guts. Most children who experience blast injury do so in a post-conflict zone. Medics who work with blast-injured children always assume that those who are brought in for treatment will be malnourished, and most will be stunted and wasted. Suddenly, we are back to the weights and measures, and not with the slow and steady pace of a humanitarian-organization research study.

All the dosages of medications that a blast-injured child is likely to need, and that are described in the textbooks, are based on normal physiological ranges. Normal children, with normal metabolisms, microbiomes and growth rates. These are no good whatsoever in the deeply abnormal world of the conflict zone. There are no formal international standards for children who are wasted *and* stunted *and* wounded. If medics don't have a scale (and it's a key piece of kit for units likely to be treating blast-injured children), they learn to pick up a child, hold it in their arms for a few seconds and guess its weight, and go with that. Since Mosul and other war zones, medics have become experienced at guessing, and an informal standard has developed: subtract two kilograms from normal weight/age ranges if the child is anything up to six years old, and four kilograms for children of six years and over.[205] Shame on us that we live in a world where such a standard is required.

Everything is complicated when it's a malnourished, blast-injured child lying on the stretcher in the medical unit. The child probably can't hear, so can't understand or respond to questions. There's a point at which they stop crying and go quiet, and this is not a good thing, especially when it comes to pain. Children gasp for air when they are frightened, and can swallow so much of it their stomachs distend, which looks like severe acute malnutrition or internal bleeding.[206] The default with internal bleeding is to operate (and lots of medics in conflict zones are surgeons, so it's a double default), but they should be really sure before opening up a malnourished child in a less than optimal medical environment, because any infection is likely to rip down what little scaffolding is left, and leave the life, like the city around them, in ruins.

And for all the complications in securing the survival of a child with blast injury, it's the life beyond survival that's going to be the real challenge, especially if it's a life that's previously been lived stunted and wasted. Let's get back to bones to understand why. Children's bones are active places, especially the long bones in their arms and legs that grow faster than those thicker bones in the trunk. They are the first bones to grow thriftily in stunting, but the mechanics of growth remain the same, and are completely different to those of adults. Long bones grow at each end, from a particular area preprogrammed to do the growing and lengthening, called the growth plate. This is not bone; it's a fairly weak form of living tissue, less strong than ligaments and tendons, and definitely not as strong as bone, nor as dense, so it doesn't show up on X-rays.

When children break something, it tends to be their growth plate, rather than the bone it has already grown, but in order to properly diagnose and treat it, usually an X-ray of both legs is taken, so any gapping caused by the break on one side can be compared to the other, ungapped side. Growth plates all over the body don't grow at a consistent rate – the ones at the knee end of the long leg-bones grow fastest of all, and don't liaise with the plates at the hip end or with their twin on the other side. Growth plates eventually stop their frantic work in puberty, triggered by hormones, and the mature leg bone becomes bone all the way to the end. Presence or absence of growth plates on a skeleton is one way for us to tell if its owner was an adult or a child. For the rest of our lives, the long bones will grow, but more slowly and not very much, and, as we age, they degrade, unless we pay attention. There is evidence from work done on children stunted by chronic inflammatory conditions, such as colitis and juvenile arthritis, that their growth plates are directly affected by the hormone imbalance caused by the condition.[207] We haven't yet determined if malnutrition-related chronic inflammation has the same effect, but we know that all stunted and wasted children still have growth plates, even if they are working overtime constantly calculating how much the bone should be growing and what energy they can use from a fluctuating store.

Until they don't. Blast injury often – usually – means limb loss. Growth plates that have been blown off don't regenerate. So the bone that is left there grows as adult bone, slowly and not much. And what is left of the limb will require, as the textbook says, close surveillance.[208] Rehab and prosthetic fit will be difficult. Amputations are complicated enough in adults, but in children the complications go to a whole other level, especially in an environment which is suboptimal for everything, including surveillance.

So the end of one limb (or more) will grow slowly and not much, and all the other growth plates keep doing their work, keenly and actively. Any prosthetic limb fitted to align with a leg or arm of a certain length will need to be replaced with another limb sooner rather than later. Try tracking patients who need this kind of surveillance through Britain's NHS – we haven't done that successfully yet, so imagine the equivalent patient displaced in a conflict or post-conflict zone. We have some sense of the pain of amputations and prosthetic use, but not much that's child specific. In life beyond survival, a quiet child is still a child with pain, just one that's got used to it because nothing much can be done. (And pain can lessen appetite.) Children grow out of their prosthetics, as they would have the shoes they should have had, again and again. Pain, refit, rehab – until puberty and the sealing of the remaining growth plates. And in the meantime, we don't understand much of what happens to the overall anatomical structure that they take into adulthood. The only in-depth studies of disordered gait in children are done by researchers into the effects of cerebral palsy, where muscle strength and volume are less than normal.[209] It's not much research, and it's done on children who grow up far away from conflict zones, but at least it's something, and we could, if we tried a little bit harder, apply its lessons to everyone who needs wasted muscle and their gait rebuilt.

And none of the above is the worst of it. Wherever it is experienced, for whatever reason, borne by whichever Horseman, malnutrition has a significant impact on cognitive development. For all the thriftiness of the human system, eventually stunting and wasting hits the human brain. Macro- and micronutrient deficiency is a significant factor in children failing to reach their development potential, especially if they are doing their growing up somewhere with inadequate cognitive stimulation. If no one regularly reads them a story, at a regular bedtime, in a place where they are well fed, warm, comfortable and likely to get untroubled sleep and good dreaming done, then they may never follow a story all the way to its end, never mind read one for themselves. The scientific term for this kind of activity is nurturing. Scientists, like those in the Prendergast Lab, know what they mean when they say it, and they explain with something approaching force that nurturing is a key component in combatting malnutrition, and that perfectly fed children can fail to thrive if no one nurtures them, so malnutrition is never, ever just about food. The Centro Internacional de la Papa has learned this lesson about nurturing too, and they encourage the farmers who participate in their programmes to put their children to play or to bed more than they put them to work.

Nurturing is a childhood-long commitment to the small domestic details of care, beginning at the beginning, because, just like the rest of the body, the brain does most of its growing in the first one thousand days. If it can't put its own scaffolding up, then connections aren't made and the owner of the brain is less likely to be able to remember, to reason, to solve problems, to understand complicated things and learn from their experiences. Just learning to be themselves becomes much more difficult without nurturing. And, additionally, stunted and wasted children have impaired behavioural development. They are less likely to explore (although if they live in a post-conflict zone, there's some advantage in that), they can be more apathetic than normally nourished children, and they are often anxious and depressed.[210] Malnourished children go to school late, and do badly when they get there, and stay for less time, and so grow up less able to contribute to the rebuilding of their society: malnutrition rips down the scaffolding and fabric of nations, just as it does with humans.

The long-term effects of blast injury make it difficult for children to be educated at all, even if the schools haven't been blown up. Blast waves can damage sight and hearing, limb loss is costly – children need expensive healthcare and may not be able to walk to school or work. A child with limb loss is a child that experiences higher levels of violence, forced marriage and bonded labour than their uninjured fellows. Children with disability, all over the world, are four times more likely to experience violence than their non-disabled peers.[211] The only thing that doesn't falter is time. Children, innocent victims of conflict, become adolescents, who grow up into adults, no longer stunted, just short, living with the cumulative effects of pain and disability for which there is no science. And somehow, as adults, they are considered less innocent, less worthy of the television appeals and news coverage. Malnourished children never learn who they are, never mind who they could be. All that potential that they are born with is simply wasted.

More than anything, that's what places like the Prendergast Lab are trying to do: stop the waste of lives. Like everyone in this book, underneath the very complicated scientific language, they have some very simple messages and dreams. They'd like to prevent the waste of lives in the first place, but prevention is very difficult, so until the day when the Horsemen are nowhere to be found, we do our best to compensate for the effects of malnutrition. We've learned a lot in the last ten years to help enable children wounded by war and famine to catch up and somehow be the human beings their cells thought they could be on the day they were born. The technical term for catching up is 'catch-up'. Stunted children don't just need to start eating properly again. Their bodies need to catch up with all the growing and development they should have been doing in the first thousand days, when life almost stopped and became about nothing much more than survival. Catch-up means a period of rapid growth, following growth inhibition, and it's a recognized scientific thing. To catch up, food and micronutrients are needed to put the scaffolding back up, to start building a normal human, and at the right time. Catch-up happens at places like the growth plate, because it's so active and keen a biomaterial. Timing is everything. The huge growth spurts that should happen in the first one thousand days of a human's life, with the accompanying, interacting hormonal message systems telling everything to get going, especially bones, don't last forever. It's a continuation of foetal growth (growth done in the womb) and it slows down naturally. So catch-up needs to occur when this first growth spurt is underway.

For those humans who live in food insecurity or famine, as in Yemen, micronutrients are part of the recipe used in the general feeding programmes that are delivered by the full spectrum of humanitarian organizations. They comprise 'a supplement of 500–1200 kcal per day, consisting of fortified blended food mixed with oil . . . in the form of an onsite meal or a dry take-home premix'.[212] So cereal wheat and soya is blended with a fortificant premix, so it's as nutritious as food can be. These blended provisions have another advantage. It's always clearly marked on the sacks that they are blends, and despite the higher nutritional quality, this makes them less valuable for resale, so they tend not to get stolen or sold on the black market (which, if they were just wheat, they would be, because wheat sells well for ready money, which is why they are planting it so frantically in Yemen) and are instead eaten by those who are hungry. They are a good, basic, readily transportable, readily distributable foodstuff. But for those with catching up to do, more is needed.

Micronutrients are given additionally, in a range of forms, in everything from properly iodized salt to tablets and syrups (and not forgetting the new nutri-dense sweet-potato variety, with extra pro-Vitamin A and enhanced iron content, developed by the Centro Internacional de la Papa). Vitamin A is put into capsules containing oils that dissolve slowly in the human system and ensure a steady dose for up to six months. They are big tablets to swallow, but go down easily and won't need topping up for a while. Children between one and four and breastfeeding mothers get the biggest ones, and babies and pregnant women get a slightly smaller version. It's similar with iodine: salt for the families and capsules for children, large doses that slowly and effectively compensate for deficiency, allowing for just one treatment per year. Iron is a little more difficult. It doesn't hang around for long in the body, so needs to be topped up regularly. Pregnant women and low-weight babies are given tablets and drops until their levels are restored, sometimes for as long as a month, and there's iron-enriched syrup for preschoolers.[213] Single-dose sachets of multiple vitamins and minerals are given to families to mix into food at home, but this assumes home, and food, and families. There are many other supplements and interventions that can be performed alongside the micronutrient programmes, but what everyone doing the intervening has always agreed on is that it all needs to take place within the first one thousand days, because otherwise it isn't effective at generating catch-up. The supplements will prevent the child becoming sicker, will mean longer intervals between infections, but they won't reverse the stunting.

Recently, though, we've begun to understand that there might be a second opportunity to catch up, when scaffolding and hormones start going up again, as the body prepares for a second, final growth spurt, in adolescence.[214] Currently, we recognize adolescence as lasting from ten to nineteen years old. We should be recognizing more that this period is every bit as vital to our development as human beings as the first thousand days. Growth in adolescence is rapid – we get about 25 per cent of our full height here – and just like the first thousand days, we need the hormonal messaging to get out there and tell our bones and interacting systems to get on with it. Our energy needs, and our need for micronutrients, are at their very highest in our whole lives at this point. Particularly in our bones. Adolescent bones are busy places. It's peak calcium-deposition time, with up to 300 milligrams a day added to our bone mass, and although the medical textbooks say that growing pains are muscle related, it's hard to imagine that bones straining to become grown-up skeletons can be achieved without us noticing. It's difficult to apply weight and height standards, because the variations in adolescents are simply too complex, but it's accepted that adolescents who experience malnutrition can become both stunted and wasted to the point at which growth stops altogether. Gender doesn't kick in as much of a distinguishing factor in stunting until puberty, and then it does. Girls begin puberty earlier, and the density of their bones is different from that of boys. Stunted girls who become pregnant in adolescence are most likely to be stunted forever, because their spare growing energy will go to their foetus, who has all that prenatal growing to do, although spare won't be enough, and stunted mothers usually mean stunted babies, who will probably go on to have more stunted babies, and all of them are more likely to be obese at some point, which can blight a life already damaged.[215] Encouraging adolescents not to get pregnant, or make other adolescents pregnant, and protecting the vulnerable against sexual violence that could lead them to be made pregnant against their will, is all helpful in the process of achieving catch-up.[216]

Just like in our first thousand days, the hormones fizzing round our bodies (if we're getting the right micronutrients) do more than just get us to grow up and out; they develop our brains, so this is where catch-up in the brain potentially happens. In adolescence, hormones in our brains refine our cognitive ability, our voluntary-control mechanisms and our executive function – the means whereby we choose our behaviour, understand our choices, make plans and see them through. So, when we're undernourished in adolescence, we're really undernourished. We'll be smaller, diminished, stunted, for the rest of our lives – and we'll probably make some really bad choices along the way. Being a teenager is hard enough, without being undernourished at the same time. What we know about adolescence that is crucial for tackling famine is that it's a time when catch-up is possible. We can get hormones to go back to doing their proper job, finishing making the child into an adult, not living thriftily just to survive. But we haven't proved it scientifically yet, because we don't know exactly why this happens.[217] All the funding for this kind of research goes into the first-thousand-days cohort (it's memorable and politically persuasive).[218] Science on adolescents isn't as appealing, especially if those adolescents are vaguely threatening-looking males. As a researcher looking into catch-up, you are more likely to get money to do animal trials (rabbits and rats) than for studies into teenage boys and malnutrition. But there are also studies that look at what is scientifically called 'markedly stunted affluent children' – patients with hormone imbalances or dietary disorders such as celiac disease. In all of these studies (and the ones with rabbits), interventions are given to supplement nutrition, and they work. What has been lost or held back is restored.

The scientists who do this work at the Prendergast Lab nodded when I read them this section, and they said predictable scientist things, like how we tend to measure catch-up with height and weight gain, but this almost certainly doesn't tell the whole story, because we don't have any equivalent measurement (yet) for proving catch-up cognition. It's scientifically very difficult to measure the effects of nurturing, even though we know it when we see it, or don't see it. So, a child may regain height or inches, but never do well at school. Or the other way around. Children may catch up intellectually, but never put the inches back on – so they go back to school smarter, but not necessarily taller.[219] The determinants of linear growth and neurodevelopment are only partly shared. So, just restoring nutrition by supplements or a proper diet will never be enough. It needs to be holistic to get the best results: nourishment all round, a good development environment, a resilient care framework, nurturing. Peace and good governance (the scientists at the Prendergast Lab always end our meetings by reminding me that these are essential components for catch-up). An external environment that is optimized for growth is the kind that is wonderful for children and terrible for Horsemen.

Here's what we do know works, for sure. It's nothing new, nothing you haven't read in the last chapter, nothing any steward won't tell you. It's nothing expensive (getting cheaper all the time), and we already do it. Vaccinations. Vaccinations prevent diseases, and prevent the complications from diseases which mean millions and millions fewer doses of antibiotics. Vaccinations are healthcare systems by other means. The science is steady on the role of immune dysfunction in malnutrition. Malnourished children get infections, which undermine their immune systems and make them more likely to get more infections, which will make them more malnourished, and eventually whatever has been built collapses. So, take infections out of the equation as much as possible. Keep the energy of a growing child where it should be, and do it as early as possible. Taking a child to get a vaccination, maintaining a medical record card, not minding the long walk or the queue at the doctors, or wiping away the tears of a child – the technical and scientific term for all of that is nurturing. So, nurture and vaccinate against everything possible, including the infections that attack the digestive system, like rotaviruses, and begin the cause and consequence of immune dysfunction in malnutrition.

At Mosul, in 2017, immediately after liberation, vaccination programmes began again. Healthcare workers were brave enough to go into the ruins of the city, despite the risks and the flies, to begin the urgent work of rebuilding its children, with food supplements for the malnourished and vaccinations for every little human being they could find. In 2019, because it is at the very heart of their remit, the WHO coordinated a huge vaccination programme against cholera in the Democratic Republic of the Congo, despite the random outbreaks of violence that could lock down cities into siege states, no one in, no one out. The healthcare workers who were responsible for delivering the programme worked not just against a background threat of violence, they worked during an Ebola outbreak, coming across other local healthcare teams delivering other vaccinations, reporting contact traces, together bringing Horsemen to a halt. More than a million children received an oral cholera vaccination (in two stages, like polio), so they are now and always will be protected from a disease which, if it didn't take their lives, would otherwise ravage their microbiome. An intact microbiome means their inflammatory mechanism will be maintained as it should be – one of those things that helps keeps them out of hospital, means they aren't given antibiotics for no good reason, and won't tie up medical staff.

So, when vaccinators return and keep going with their vaccinations in the face of local violence or global pandemics, they are supporting local healthcare systems by other means. Vaccinations don't just prevent millions and millions of unnecessary doses of antibiotics and so slow down antibiotic resistance. They also have 'beneficial non-specific effects' (that's what hope sounds like when scientists say it).[220] We vaccinate against specific infections, but we are increasingly finding that the beneficial effects of the vaccine go far beyond its targets. The BCG vaccine is used against TB and leprosy. Like all vaccines, it trains the immune system to be ready for these specific infections. The BCG vaccine 'shocks' the whole innate immune system, so it's ready for more than just the specified fight. Children who have had the BCG vaccination have generally stronger immune responses, and better overall resistance to disease. It doesn't work with all possible diseases. During 2020, there was talk of the BCG vaccination preventing children from contracting COVID, but it was only ever talk, and it distracted from the other beneficial non-specific general effects. Vaccinations very specifically benefit haemoglobin levels – the red part of blood, strengthened by iron, that transports oxygen around the body, and energy, so haemo-globin is a good biomarker for overall well-being. A vaccinated child has higher-quality haemoglobin concentrations than an unvaccinated one, before iron tablets have even come into it. The confirmation of these findings wasn't the result of an expensive randomized control trial. No new labs had to be built, or significant investments made. The study was done by looking back over the vaccination cards of 368,450 children in countries where they were at risk of stunting, when they were brought in for routine health-clinic visits. There were variables, because there always are, but the message from the study was clear. Vaccinations are good for everyone. The balance is working in favour of the human: a small action on one side delivers huge effects on the other, cheaply and easily bought.

A caveat: timing is essential. Vaccines need to be given early – well within the first-thousand-days marker – for the non-specific beneficial effects to happen. Pneumonia, part of the RSV lower respiratory tract virus family, takes up residence in the respiratory tract of children before they are two, and so, for the vaccine to be effective, it needs to get there first, so the immune system is ready to work.[221] And so far, it isn't every vaccine that has the extra non-specific effects, and it can depend on the mechanism of the dose itself. We don't know which component of the vaccination actually spurs on the beneficial effects beyond immunity, and it seems to work best with injectables, rather than oral vaccines.

But we do know it goes the other way, too. Children who are unvaccinated, who get conditions like measles, suffer the wrong kind of shock to their innate immune system from the virus which undermines it, possibly weakening their system for their entire life-time, wherever they live, no matter how much they get to eat.[222] In children malnourished from before birth, the effects of the vaccines may take a little longer, and the children will need to be fed prop-erly for them to kick in, and the vaccines may need to be given in different forms or more times. But these children in particular tell us one of the most interesting things of all about the effects of vac-cination: the way they have been designed, and the way they work, is effective even in immune systems that may have been born weak and would otherwise be thought to be faltering, perhaps not even strong enough to respond to a vaccine, but they are. Children are more resilient than we think, in ways that we are only just beginning to understand. We now know that vaccines facilitate catch-up in the immune system, if they are given at the right time and in the right format. We understand some of the genetic mechanism at work in the process, but not all of it. Some science catch-up is to be done in the meantime, while real-life things get on with their work.[223]

Here's a really sustainable development goal that we can realize once the science has caught up: 'the adjustment of current vacci-nation strategies in order to support the optimal maturation of the immune system'. A child whose immune system has been optimized is a child that can withstand lower respiratory tract infection, who may never need a prophylactic antibiotic or doses of antibiotics that don't work anymore, and who might have more of a chance of growing up to be who they always should have been, even if it's in a conflict zone. A child who may one day help negotiate or dis-cover a draw, against any given Horseman. So, every time a child is vaccinated, they step up and join the line around the world, either clutching a slightly sore arm or proudly showing their left-hand little finger, where the nail has been marked with a blue felt pen to indicate they've had a vaccination in drop form. When the rider of the black horse is forced to a stop, the draw – the balancing of his scale – is achieved with nurturing and potatoes and vaccinations. All things that are simply taught and grown, and are cheap. Get them all going in the right places, sustain them, and we really can and will save our world.

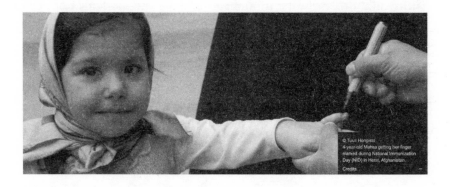

© Tuuli Hongisto.
4-year-old Mahsa getting her finger marked during National Immunization Day (NID) in Herat, Afghanistan.
Credits

In 2018, if War and Famine had tried to sneak back into Mosul down some of its remaining narrow, shadowed streets, they would have been beaten back by the sight of another very simple foodstuff. In January, a year after liberation, the historian at Mosul did a survey of what was on sale in the town's restored marketplaces and shops. He found honey, lots of it.[224] And the beekeepers of Nineveh province who had made it, eight hundred of them, who had returned to their land after the ISIS winter and had brought their hives with them, had, in that year, made 48,000 kilogram of honey, which was now for sale across Iraq, but especially in the markets of their home city (which have already been rebuilt as a priority under the UNESCO programme to #Revive the Spirit of Mosul).[225] The sight of the jars of honey meant many things (honey, in and of itself, never a bad thing). It meant that the agricultural ecosystem was being restored, despite the destruction and the oil spills and the toxic remnants of occupation and the blood of liberation. The land was recovering enough to support plants that could support bee colonies, and the natural farming cycle of Nineveh was back in the hands of people who respected it. It meant the sounds of the city had returned to a steady noisy normal, without explosions or heavy vehicles thundering by, so bees flew without fear, and the keepers tended them without fear during the day. The bees will need care. Water supplies are still low and this could affect crop yields. But Mosul bees are tough. Wherever they fled to during the war, they survived somehow and then they came back, unstressed enough to make record amounts of honey, and livings for many. Hope in a jar, in yoghurt, in tea, licked from a spoon by a child who had perhaps never known what sweetness really meant before that moment. There are beekeepers in the line, eight hundred of them at least, hive smokers at their feet, just back from market, in Mosul.

DEATH

'And behold a pale horse: and his name that sat on him was Death.'

Revelation 6:8

I have been asked a surprising amount of times if I have a favourite Horseman.[226] Perhaps even more surprisingly, I do, and it's this one. For almost everyone whose work I have described in this book up to this point, death is a failure. It is what happens when treatment or research or liberation doesn't happen in time, and human beings are lost. They learn if they can, look away and move on. But beyond this point, the line still holds, and the best way to see how it is secured is from the point of view of the pale rider. The line he sees is strong. It's full of human beings who have chosen to stand for the dead as both their first response and their life's work. I don't think I was expecting to find such commitment in such a place. Without focusing on the pale rider, without following his steady, simple gaze, I would have missed it, and missed the opportunity to show the line in its full, extraordinary entirety, all the way around our world.

Holding the line against Death is one of our most ancient human instincts. Our first response is to secure a name for the person who has died, and a place where they can be laid to rest and mourned. Across our religions and myths, humans account for those they have outlived, even if it's a strange or dangerous thing for them to do.[227] After murdering his brother Abel, Cain is ordered by his god to bury him, and then is sent, marked, into exile. The family, friends and followers of Jesus entomb his body, even though there are Roman soldiers everywhere in Jerusalem, on the lookout. To retrieve Hector's body so it can receive proper funeral rites, Priam walks out of Troy, straight into the mass of besieging Greek forces, to 'get down on my knees and do what must be done/And kiss Achilles' hand, the killer of my son'.[228] As in Homer's Troy, so in Socrates' Thebes. Antigone chooses to stand and speak for her slain brother, no matter that it will cost her own life to do so. From the stone amphitheatres of ancient Greece to Solferino and the sites of catastrophe in today's real world, her words ring simple and clear: 'the dead have rights'.[229]

But what happens to that human instinct when the numbers of dead overwhelm the living? Who speaks for them when there is almost no one else left standing? In our time, we can give something like an answer. On 26 December 2004, one Horseman surveyed the backwash of what used to be an island seashore, foam and debris streaming over the hooves of his pale horse, up to its flanks in churn, after a giant three-part tsunami had passed over Sumatra and the Andaman Islands in Indonesia, through to the ocean beyond. It left over 170,000 dead human beings in its wake. The tsunami did its killing quickly, in less than a single hour. And beyond the dead were at least 500,000 survivors, gasping for breath as they clung to life in their almost eradicated world.

There were no other Horsemen involved. The cause was an earthquake, deep out at sea (exact coordinates: 3.30 N, 95.78 E). Earthquakes occur at the points where the tectonic plates that make up our planet meet and move. We tend to think of them as shaking, but earthquake motion is crashing, scraping and rupturing. When the plates move, stress occurs, and if one side of the plate is weaker than the other, the rock ruptures, and the rupture spreads until the stress lessens or it meets a rock strong enough to withstand its force. On 26 December, the rupture occurred along the Indo-Australian plate and the Eurasian plate, thirty metres below the surface of the Indian Ocean. Seismologists now think it was probably multiple small ruptures, where pressure had been building up for some time, cracking out along any and all weak points, eventually coming together as one giant event. Officially, quakes in Chile in 1960 and Alaska in 1965 have slightly higher designations, because they were measurable. But the rupture that exploded out along the plate at the bottom of the Indian Ocean in 2004 was so big, it went unmeasurably 'off-scale'. This exact phrase was used by one of the world's leading seismologists in his *Philosophical Transactions A* report to the Royal Society of London that same year. *Phil Trans A* covers the physical sciences, including the specialist geological fields of earthquake and volcano study. The Royal Society was the first to define these new categories of scholarship in the eighteenth century. It packed members off to study volcano craters and quake sites in places such as Etna, Vesuvius and Stromboli, and published their findings and drawings in the journal, if they got back safely. Despite almost three centuries of seismology and volcanology, and the new Earth science of plate tectonics, some events still defy categorization.[230]

The reason we have a clear idea of what happened is because, six months before the Sumatra–Andaman earthquake cracked open the world, the Global Seismographic Network went live. The Global Seismographic Network is the part of a line all around the world that goes under the ocean and across mountains and up into the sky above us, and it monitors all possible seismic vibrations across planet Earth, no matter how slight or mighty. In June 2004, it had 136 out of 152 intended stations up and running, from the South Pole to Siberia, and from the Amazon basin to the Pacific Ocean (they are all operational now). In its earliest form, it looked for nuclear explosions as well as earthquakes, and it used dial-up telephone access to report its findings. Now, it uses the best broadband possible (which it calls very-broadband), and in a non-specific beneficial effect, just like the BCG vaccination, when its broadband was taken to some of its most remote stations, it also established internet infrastructure in places that hadn't really had it before, and might have remained disconnected for a long time, because no one else thought to connect them (like Pitcairn Island and remotest Mongolia).

Of all the surveillance systems around the world listening out for earthquakes, it was the GSN's that was the biggest in 2004, and its data told us that what happened 250 kilometres off the Indonesian Banda Aceh coast was the worst seismic event ever experienced in human history. The rupture zone was longer than any other earthquake ever recorded. The fractures and cracks spread along a 1,300-kilometre line – an 808-mile split in the Earth's crust – many times longer than anything recorded before. The rupture lines travelled along the fault at about 2.5 kilometres per hour from their various starting points. The entire event lasted 600 seconds (seismologists measure everything in seconds, but to the rest of us, this is about ten minutes).[231] Out of sight, thirty metres below the ocean surface, we'd have to use the best CGI to even imagine what that would have looked like, but we didn't have to wait long to see its effects.

A huge area of seabed deformed, and an even huger area (a trillion tons) of ocean water was displaced. The only way for this kind of energy to disperse across an ocean is in the form of wavelengths, very long and high, which are pushed on out until they eventually dissipate, or something stronger, like land, gets in the way. This phenomenon is known as a tsunami. Earthquakes that cause tsunamis (i.e. undersea ones) are said to be tsunamigenic, and the process is known as 'exciting' a tsunami. On 26 December 2004, the earthquake excited three huge tsunami waves, which spread out across the Indian Ocean and took between fifteen and thirty minutes to make nearest landfall. There was no warning. There could not have been. There were no precursors or foreshocks that would indicate to the relevant authorities to expect anything. No matter how much money we spend (so it wasn't a question of under-resourcing), we currently don't have any technology that enables us to accurately predict earthquakes, although it's what those using the data from the Global Seismographic Network are ultimately working towards.

Those sentinels of the GSN can watch, can measure, but cannot yet warn of anything but imminence.

The nearest landfall was Aceh, the province at the northernmost tip of the island of Sumatra. Aceh is relatively flat, made of coastal plain – much of it tidal – that supports shrimp and fish ponds. Sumatra itself is a long thin island, following the shape of the fault line that shattered on 26 December. The first thing the coastal residents of Aceh province registered about the catastrophe speeding across the ocean towards them at 800 kilometres per hour was something like the sound of a very large aircraft overhead. If they were awake, they probably looked up to see what it was, rather than over and out to sea. Seismic events very rarely sound ominous. In 2010, a very large earthquake devastated the island of Haiti, but at the moment that it struck, it sounded to everyone like a really big truck going by, until their houses fell down around them and they realized it must be something else.[232] Aceh has rivers and beach ridges, dunes and levees which shape its coastline. These would have some mitigating effect as the waves hit, but not much. Tsunamis aren't like normal sea waves, so they cannot be surfed. There is no wave face, so there would be nothing for a surfboard to grip on to, and they move from top to sea floor, so no duck-diving is possible to get away from them, as a surfer might normally do. Tsunamis don't break. They move just as they are, as huge areas of displaced water, in a solid block, a turbulent concrete debris-laden block. It is energy in its most brutal visible form. A wave and a block at the same time.

The energy in the block is much more powerful than that in a breaking wave, and it is irresistible until it begins to disperse. It took four kilometres of Banda Aceh territory to disperse the energy of the tsunami on 26 December, and, as oceanographers now understand, it's usually the second wave-block that does the most damage (it draws energy from the first wave as it makes landfall, doubling up). If the first wave-block was nine metres high, it is likely that the second was fifteen metres higher than normal sea level. The energy it bore from top to bottom was savage. It stripped bark from trees, miles inland. It swept away whole buildings, the only sign they had ever been there a footprint of tiled flooring, itself deeply scoured and scratched as the wave passed over (and there is a particular verb that describes this action: wave scour). If there was a third, we don't have much information about it. Its progress was lost in the brutal chaos unfurling across Banda Aceh, now under four or five metres of water. Even when the inundation slowly began to drain away, it didn't recede completely. The shoreline is now 1.5 kilometres from where it was on the evening of 25 December.

And in that inundation, along 800 kilometres of coastline, lay the 170,000 dead. In the worst-damaged areas, a quarter of the population was lost, including a third of the children under seven. The technical description that would later be applied to this loss is 'an event of immense mortality'.[233] Some villages were simply wiped away by the water – every human, every tree, every sign that they had ever existed, gone – only battered brown earth remaining.[234] In some villages, only men were left, and only some of those – the ones who could swim, who were strong enough or lucky enough to find something to cling to in exhaustion, after they had gone back and back and back again, trying in vain to rescue their families. Everyone in Aceh province lost someone – a friend, a family member. At least 10,000 children lost one parent, and almost 5,000 were orphaned. Entire kinship networks were destroyed. Those that were left stood among destruction worse than anything war can conceive. Later, 1.3 trillion cubic metres of debris would be recorded as having been cleared (one cubic metre of tsunami debris would have weighed about one tonne; by comparison, Mosul has recorded eleven million tonnes of debris cleared from its streets). In Aceh, their world had gone in less than an hour, and as the evening of 26 December fell, the satellites on orbits that passed above the island recorded almost half as much light from the region most affected as there should have been.[235]

During the day, the death toll rose around the Indian Ocean, as the tsunami hit Sri Lanka (35,000 killed), India (18,000 killed) and Thailand (8,000 killed). In every country, this was beyond mass casualty preparations. There was nowhere on the coastline of the Indian Ocean that was not affected, as the tsunami spread in all directions from its epicentre. Heading north-east, it hit the Malaysian coast, and up to Thailand and Myanmar. In its midfield, 1,600 miles from the epicentre, to the north-west, it hit a long line down the Indian coast and the island of Sri Lanka. Straight west, an hour later, the wave struck the Maldives, which were low lying then, and are even more so now. There were fewer deaths, here, but the tsunami smashed through buildings and livelihoods just the same. Five thousand kilometres from the epicentre, three hours later, waves reached East Africa, where the wave-block killed 300 people in the coastal lowlands of Somalia and devastated the local fishing industry, which was already suffering the effects of piracy in the region.[236] Kenya, Tanzania and Madagascar all felt its effects, and tourists in Oman wondered why the sea lapping up to their pristine beaches was so murky, and full of garbage labelled in a faraway language.

The last accountings were done on Yemeni territory: the island archipelago of Socotra, where unique relic species of plants called dragon trees (*Dracaena cinnabari*) grow, which bleed red if you cut into their trunks. Inundations of up to six metres hit low-lying southern areas, less elsewhere, and damaged ports, stone-built houses, fishing fleets. One death happened after a seven-year-old boy ran to catch a fish lying on the exposed sea floor during the drawdown that always happens before the wave-block strikes.[237] Twenty-five hours later, the tsunami's waves were still triggering pressure gauges in other oceans. The detectors of the Global Seismographic Network and all the other seismology monitoring technology equipment across the world, wherever they were, recorded at least a 1 per cent rise in vibration levels due to the earthquake's impact. The whole surface of our planet had been moved. There have been other earthquakes since, and they have been tsunamigenic, and some of them (like the one that hit the coast of Japan in 2011 and caused the Fukushima nuclear plant to melt down) have had serious consequences, but nothing – repeat, nothing – on the scale of Indonesia in 2004.

And almost all of the dying had been done by the first nightfall. Across the world, the cries from the survivors resounded, despite the wave having scoured away telephone and power cables, mobile-phone towers and generating stations. The UN saw the wave and called for force to meet force, for huge emergency resources to be

deployed immediately. Its Office for the Coordination of Humanitarian Affairs (OCHA, who we have met before in this book, at
Mosul) was summoned. As per their remit, they called a meeting
'to mobilize and coordinate the humanitarian response for optimal
efficiency, effectiveness and speed'. They instigated a global Flash
Appeal for money to pay for it. As the rest of the world woke to the
news, time zone by time zone, the Flash Appeal worked. The money
rolled in, an inundation of its own – over a billion US dollars, by
the end – although it took a while to connect resource with need,
because in addition to scouring away cables and power lines, there
were no roads, no bridges, no infrastructure, and nothing looked
like it did on the maps that had been made before the morning of
26 December and the wave-block of water that swept all before it.
It would be ten days and nights before contact was made with every
last surviving community in Aceh.

From Sumatra to Socotra and back again. Across the ocean in Aceh,
the next morning, the pale horse and its rider stand watching the
aftermath as the water calms around them, unconcerned by its floating
filth and shocking cargo. Their presence should remind us that, to
understand Aceh, we must remember its dead, the immensity of the
mortality, because only from there can we fully understand what came
next. The first thing to grasp is that there is nowhere on Earth that has
the capacity to deal with as many dead as there were in the aftermath of
the tsunami in Aceh. It's what really marks natural disasters out from
the man-made kind. Aceh joins a select group of modern-era disasters,
where planetary forces have ripped into whole populations with instant
brutality. In 1970, it is estimated (because they never really knew) that

between 300,000 and 500,000 human beings were killed in a sudden night-time storm surge in the Bay of Bengal. The Tangshan earthquake in China, in 1976, had 242,000 casualties killed, there and then, as the earth shook and gaped. This is not like the counting and posting of the dead after battles, or the uneven creep of death rates in epidemics and pandemics. It is something very different: immense numbers of dead, suddenly, and then no more. Because it happened in the twenty-first century, with its array of technological witnesses, Aceh is the single event of immense mortality that we know best.

After we see the dead, we should see the local people who survived, who had to make the first response to so much destruction, often before they knew if anyone would come to save them or to help them, or how many survivors there were, or if this was the end of the whole world, or just theirs. In every moment of their first response, searching for the missing became discovery of the dead. In accordance with those oldest of human instincts – and just as it had happened at Solferino – in the heat and humidity of the morning of the next day, the people of Aceh organized themselves into groups and began to dig to bury the dead around them, to return those who had come from the soils and sands of Aceh to the same ground. Except it was not the same ground. Layers of deposited mud and silt and salt water had changed the soil composition into an entirely new ground beneath their feet. Gravel had mixed with sand, and the matted rags of farm crops and grasslands were already rotting. Debris had smashed into what had once been fields and dunes. Levees had gone, and no one knew when the tide would come in, or where it would come up to, or where they could safely and securely dig.

This is the first lesson learned from Aceh. Anywhere in the world where such an immensity of death was experienced would face the same essential basic problem: land is necessary for burials. The dead have to be buried quickly, preferably in a single layer, and their identity recorded, in case they need to be exhumed or moved. To do that, there needs to be enough land. Government land that has been officially designated and marked on maps is the first assumption. The very idea of what was and wasn't government land in Aceh was complicated, so no one knew for sure where to start, and mostly there was no one to ask. As hours passed, numbers, heat, humidity and matters of faith made rapid burial the only option. Mass graves were dug wherever they could be, either very large – some containing 60,000 bodies or more – or very small, a few families' worth, but in the wrong place, too near or sometimes inside surviving villages.

There's a graph of how many bodies were buried in Aceh, day by day, and the achievement by a shattered survivor population is somehow, and I'm not sure I know the right words for this, extraordinarily impressive. On the first day, they buried 3,000 people. On the second day, another 3,000, and on the third day, close to 5,000. Burial of all the dead was completed by February 2005, although after a few days, the survivors had help from the Indonesian army, primarily, who arrived to coordinate and complete the process.[238] It was the Indonesian army that plotted the graph, because they contacted everyone who dug, who found something that worked as a body bag, who didn't walk away and hope that someone else would do the work, who took a photo or kept something that might help later with identification, who became part of a body-recovery team before they even knew what the name meant, and who stood in the line each day and held together their shaken world.

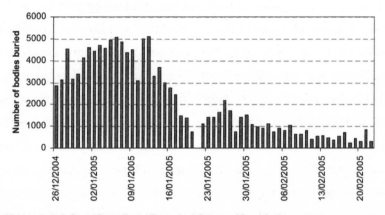

Note: Districts include Pantai Barat, Pantai Timur, Aceh Besar and Band Aceh.
Source: Badan Koordinasi Nasional Penanggulangan Bencana Dan Penanganan Pengungsi (BAKORNAS PBP)

Eventually, specialist teams in dealing with what is officially known as the management of the dead started to arrive in the wake of the wave. But they didn't get to Aceh for a long time, even if we think they did. In much of the rest of the world, when we try to understand the tsunami of 2004, the images we have in our head are not from Indonesia, they are from the other shores along the Indian Ocean that were affected, especially Thailand. There had been foreign tourists there for Christmas on the beach, and foreign workers in the hotels, and when the world woke up on 26 December, Thailand had a unique tsunami-casualty cohort. Eight thousand, two hundred people had been killed instantly, and 2,400 of those were of forty-one different nationalities. The families and governments from each of the forty-one countries across the shaken planet wanted their own identified and brought back home as quickly as possible. To do that, they called the provider of first resort when the dead need identification and repatriation across national borders: Interpol.

Interpol's full name is the International Criminal Police Organization, and they are an IGO (an intergovernmental organization, like the UN) that is made up of member countries – 194, in Interpol's case. Their mandate is to help police in all of their member countries to work together to make the world a safer place. So they fight crime, increasingly in cyberspace, and they help countries investigate terrorist incidents. Interpol is about establishing identities, securing resolution, wherever something happens. So when a country has experienced a terrorist attack, Interpol can help them investigate the perpetrators and bring them to justice. Where that terrorist attack has damaged national emergency procedures to the point that identifying and managing dead foreign nationals is burdensome, it's Interpol who steps in. We travel more and more, and further away from home, and if something happens to us there, whether it's a crime or an accident or a natural disaster, then our families at home need a place to start to find out what has happened to us. Mostly, that starting place would be Interpol, who have at their disposal the Interpol twenty-four-hour Command and Coordination Centre, in Lyon, France, and a Global Complex for Innovation, in Singapore. Their communications network is impeccable, duty rosters and language resources are maintained at a consistently excellent level, and they stay across the latest scientific developments in genetics, imaging, physiology and logistics, all as they relate to forensics and

disaster-victim identification (which they call DVI). They understand that what they are aiming for, in addition to supporting any
criminal procedures, is healing and rebuilding, identification and
resolution. The latest human capabilities are aligned with the oldest
human instincts.

So it was Interpol that assembled 2,000 international forensic and
police experts, and got them on flights to Thailand as soon as possible
in the new year of 2005. Slotting quickly into the hotel rooms now
empty of tourists who had all flown home, the teams brought in
portable refrigerated mortuary units, which turned into purpose-built
facilities connected to DNA labs beyond Thailand, from China
to Australia, who helped process what would eventually be digital
records in excess of eighty gigabytes of data. They set up offices where
records and findings could be reconciled, and they grouped together
all the different national resources into one Thai-based command
and control structure, while keeping up clear, regular communication
with national governments. In Britain, the Foreign Office had issued
a phone number for concerned relatives to call. By the end of the
first day of the phone lines being opened, they had received 38,000
calls, reporting 22,000 people missing, and it was up to those on the
ground in Thailand to process this information. (Eventually, it would
be determined that the final death toll of UK citizens in Thailand
was 147.) And although Interpol's mandate was to find the foreign
nationals unaccounted for, they worked as best they could with Thai
authorities searching to identify their own citizens.

Interpol had known Thailand would be a long, difficult mission,
and it was. Working in hot and heavy hazmat suits to prevent con-

tamination, with bodies stored in close-to-capacity cold facilities, was always going to be a struggle. Their teams found and identified (very nearly almost) everyone they were looking for by February 2006, a year after they arrived, and then the last of them, from both sides of the mortuary table, went home. It had been, in their own words, a situation where global theories and practices of disaster-victim identification management and identification procedures had been tested to limits not previously encountered. And they were the limits of dealing with Thailand's tsunami catastrophe, a mass casualty and mass mortality event by almost any standards. Except, on the other side of the Indian Ocean, where Aceh lay in ruins, new standards had been scoured into the land, with no foreign nationals numbered among their dead, and so no Interpol or Interpol equivalent – a catastrophic event beyond any limit.

The reality of Aceh in those first few weeks after the wave can be seen in the reports that were written afterwards, although, as none of them were written with the urgent clarity of *The Mosul Trauma Response*, it can be hard to get at the human detail. The humanitarian agencies that had attended first the OCHA meeting, and then in Aceh itself, formed the Tsunami Evaluation Coalition. Their first review was written 'with the humanitarian professional in mind', in 2007.[239] Beware anything written with the humanitarian professional in mind, because it will be full of jargon and acronyms, none of which will stick, so even just a few years after publication, it will read as if it is in old computer code. Almost smothered under whatever phraseology was current in 2007 was some serious self-criticism. There was no UN-country team close by, so just getting into the right bit of the Indonesian archipelago was difficult. And Christmas was being celebrated in much of the world, and it turned out that OCHA didn't work very well at Christmas, because so many of its staff were on holiday, so the people left manning the phones were young and inexperienced, and there was almost no one who spoke the relevant languages, so coordination with those struggling on the ground was difficult.[240] There were questionable terms of reference (which I think is humanitarian-report language for 'no one really knew what they were doing') and OCHA staff were short of petty cash in what is termed 'the acute phase of the crisis', during the first two weeks, even though the money for the Flash Appeal was pouring in. What is missing from the reports is any substantial material on what was the biggest challenge to first responders: the management of the dead (although they did include some mortality pie charts).

Interpol had its own *Tsunami Evaluation Working Group Report*, written for itself, for the world, and in the service of all those who were unrecoverable from the immense mortality of Aceh. Forensic scientists are used to looking death in the face. In their report, they looked across the ocean at the rider of the pale horse and did not flinch from understanding what he really meant. The report started with the acknowledgement that Thailand had not been Indonesia, and that, no matter that they had been tested to limits not previously encountered, whatever came next, it would need to fit anywhere and everywhere, no matter what. 'The present thinking for a massive death toll situation is not fit for purpose in delivering our principles of forensic identification and the South East Asian Tsunami of 2004 tells us it is in urgent need of revision.'[241]

Then they did what few similar organizations ever really do: the Interpol working group began to work. They were already a key component in an organizational process that was open and ready to implement their recommendations. Humanitarian Forensic Action (HFA) had begun more than twenty years before the tsunami smashed its way through Aceh. Their choice of name is not incidental. It is the science of forensics, aligned with the principles of humanitarianism, delivered by people who learn by doing. Not Humanitarian Forensic Science, not Humanitarian Forensic Alliance or Cluster – Humanitarian Forensic *Action*.

Humanitarian Forensic Action began in Argentina, in 1984, in a newly restored democracy with a population trying to come to terms with its past. A group called the Grandmothers of the Plaza de Mayo sought help from anyone they could to find their relatives who had gone missing or been killed during military rule (from 1976 to 1983). Many of them believed they had grandchildren out there somewhere, stolen from murdered parents and raised beyond their families. They wanted help with identification and resolution. They wanted, if possible, to get them back. They didn't yet trust the institutions of their own government, so in 1984, the first meeting took place between an international delegation of forensic scientists and what is always called collectively 'the Grandmothers'. The international delegation of scientists didn't speak much Spanish, and the Grandmothers had little English, so they found a young medical student, Morris Tidball-Binz – who had very little interest in forensics, but did speak English – to attend the meeting and to translate. The Grandmothers had two questions for the scientists, as technical as they were emotional: could the group identify children stolen from their original families, and could they identify bodies buried in mass graves? And the answer from the international delegation was yes, to both.

And so they did. From that first meeting came an Argentina-based forensic team with leadership and guidance from across the (at the time, relatively small) forensic world. Everyone learned fast. Forensics in this space had to be multidisciplinary: anthropology, archaeology, pathology, fingerprint analysis, dental analysis (odontology), genetics. Some of the questions were new and seemed hard, but were, in reality, easy and important to answer. Forensic haemogenetics (genetic markers found in blood samples) could distinguish grand-paternity indicators as well as those of paternity; it could be used to identify grandchildren as well as children. The Grandmothers offered themselves as scientific evidence, rolling up their sleeves to give blood samples in the knowledge that the young people in white coats in the laboratory finally offered them the certainty denied them everywhere else. In less than a year, the forensic results supported a successful court case to establish the true identity of a stolen baby girl, and to restore her to her original family. The scientists didn't just work case by case. A genetic databank was set up, so the group's work could continue. The leaders of what is now called the Argentine Forensic Anthropology Team think they'll still be using the databank in 2050 to find and account for all of Argentina's missing children and their families.

Beyond Argentina, the process underlying Humanitarian Forensic Action grew. Interpol had been the first organization to use forensics to solve international crime, and they always saw the potential for using forensics as a resource for the service of all humanity.²⁴² It wasn't just their material assets that could be put to work; Interpol provided the first ethical structures for humanitarian forensics, based on international law. Interpol has its own General Assembly, which, like that of the UN, is its supreme governing body, comprising representatives from each of its member countries. It meets once a year and each session lasts around four days. Its purpose is to ensure that Interpol's activities correspond to the needs of its member countries, and also to provide a forum to debate wider issues in its work, to secure identification and resolution. In 1996, its General Assembly met to define, propose and ratify a legal framework for a new kind of humanitarian principle: the universal right to be recognized after death. Just as Antigone had declared, sometime around 441 BCE: the dead have rights. There had been provisions within international law for the dignified treatment of the dead, but they weren't quite solid enough for anyone at Interpol. After 1996, they were. When HFA forensic humanitarians tell their own history (which they do really well), the ratification of the universal right to be recognized after death is the key turning point. It's the point at which the pale rider looks up and realizes his part of the line is actually built on very strong foundations, and much better staffed than he ever thought possible.

But there was still a way to go. Forensic scientists worked with international investigators seeking to hold the perpetrators of atrocities in the former Yugoslavia to account. These were primarily criminal investigations, and the scientists found it frustrating not to be able to use their resources and access to also provide information for the families of those killed, as part of the same process. So pressure grew for an institutional infrastructure to support the legal and humanitarian principle. Forensic scientists began reminding everyone, but especially humanitarians, that international humanitarian law and the Geneva Conventions made not only significant provision for the respect and protection of the dead, but also for resolution for their families. Specifically, Additional Protocol 1 to the Geneva Conventions, Article 23, which states: 'Families have the right to know the fate of their relatives.'[243] The dead *and* their families have rights. And although the first priority of humanitarian provision would always be for the living, sometimes there would be an equally urgent need to manage the dead. As it stood, however, the humanitarian agencies had little to offer, even though it was clearly their mandate. In Geneva, eventually, people began to listen, and to hear echoes of Henri Dunant in the words of the forensic scientists. In 2003, the ICRC finally began to recognize the concept of humanity after life, and established its own forensic unit, the first of its kind in the humanitarian world, under the leadership of Dr Morris Tidball-Binz, the young medical student who had translated for the Grandmothers when they asked their questions of the international delegation of scientists who came to Argentina. Now grown into a professor, he spends every working moment developing the concept and practice of Humanitarian Forensic Action.

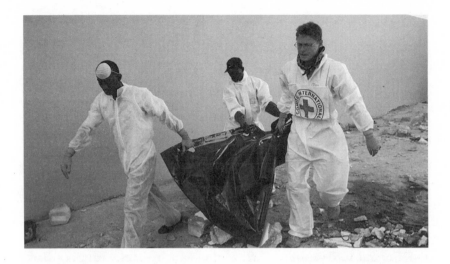

Morris Tidball-Binz, right, the head of the ICRC forensic unit, together with staff from the Central Mortuary in Port-au-Prince, Haiti, carrying a victim of the January 2010 earthquake to the morgue for identification and release to family members.

Between 2003 and 2018, the forensics unit morphed into the ICRC's Missing Persons Project – a rare example in the humanitarian world of a really great name. A missing person is a phrase we all know, and they might be lost or dead, but either way their fate is unknown. Among its staff are forensic specialists in medicine, pathology, anthropology, odontology, archaeology and criminalistics. The Project is about resolution, and it builds on forensic science, but it also seeks to understand better ways to connect with the family or community groups from which the missing person originates – by developing good working relationships, trust, dialogue. Its leaders want families to feel that everything possible has been done, and in a serious and professional way. Sometimes where resolution isn't going to be possible, then participation in the process can also be healing. Taking part, understanding, recognizing the families as primary stakeholders – working for the dead is also working for the living. Humanitarian Forensic Action, as part of the Missing Persons Project and in other organizations beyond it, now comprises scientific expertise, international law, human rights and a well-staffed and stocked international HQ (two, now: Geneva and Lyon, for its Interpol component) with absolute clarity about their mission. Today, the ICRC has formal codification of how international humanitarian law relates to humanity after life, because of HFA and the patience of its founders to hold the line.[244] It has given a space for focus, for certainty and understanding about the management of the dead, which never existed before. In 2018, the *International Review of the Red Cross* dedicated its first issue to the theme of 'The Missing'. Articles included an interview with Morris Tidball-Binz (who dedicated the piece to María Isabel Chorobik de Mariani, founder and first president of the Grandmothers, who had died that year, having lived long enough to see her work realized), as well as a piece, from one of the leading scholars of Islamic law and jurisprudence, on 'Management of the dead from the Islamic law and international humanitarian law perspectives: Considerations for humanitarian forensics'.[245]

HFA takes the line past the pale rider, fortifying as it goes. In 2017, members of the Argentine team joined the ICRC Missing Persons Project in the Falkland Islands, to assist with the identification of Argentine soldiers buried as unknowns in the cemetery after the war in the South Atlantic in 1982. One hundred and six families found resolution – much too late, but better than never. Tidball-Binz led the group, and said:

> Personally this case has convinced me of the importance of the deceased for their families, their communities and their countries. Argentina and the United Kingdom are now in peace, with full diplomatic relations, but this issue still is controversial. Although it could not be the objective in itself, the fact the dead can rest in peace, is a fundamental step to build confidence among nations.[246]

The blood-red Horseman halted, from a little more peace for families, to a little more peace in the world. We didn't know forensics had that superpower, but through Humanitarian Forensic Action, it does. Most of us know what we know about forensics from the global television franchise *CSI*. It perhaps unhelpfully raised expectations of technology in the space. Morris Tidball-Binz talks about it as 'a television show [that gave] forensics a trendy profile', but he never has to explain what his department does anymore, and before *CSI* that was complicated. From classical Greek drama to a high-budget television drama, it's all part of the same process whereby our humanity is secured and understood after our death. At Mosul, as the battle thundered on, the historian asked that the liberators of the city look for the mass graves dug by ISIS for their victims, and 'please find those graves and re-bury them in dignity again'.

Returning to the 2006 Interpol report from their work after the tsunami had struck Thailand, we can see that it contains lots of practical points and reminders, of which the most recognizable in our everyday lives is: remember to back up your computers. In one part of the Thailand report, the authors say what a miracle it was that those eighty gigabytes of data weren't lost, because there were no backups, not nightly or weekly or ever (and this was pre-cloud). But their main learning, for themselves and everyone who was a part of the Humanitarian Forensic Action process, was the meaning and reality of immense mortality: there will never be enough money or enough time or new technology in the world to deal with so many dead; their time as humanitarians was better spent thinking about what could be done, on the first or the next day, then and there.[247] Time was wasted if it was spent focusing on the technology they didn't have, or should have, or that might arrive, but never in sufficient quantities. As Morris Tidball-Binz puts it: 'The best is the enemy of the possible.' This is where HFA are truly, inspiringly radical about the future. They focus on the survivors, not as being simply the recipients of aid and humanitarian assistance, but as being key to what happens in the immediate aftermath of the immense mortality, because it's happening to them. And they have worked out how they, as forensic scientists, can help survivors then and there, where they stand, supporting what's possible as they watch the bodies of those who didn't make it wash towards them on the tide.

They've begun by redefining survivorship and have adapted the designation of 'first responders' to the context of mass or immense mortality. We think about first responders as those who have special training, usually paramedics, who are summoned to scenes of catastrophe to try to save lives. Forensic humanitarians think of them more directly: they are the people who have to respond to death, first and foremost. So now Forensic Humanitarian Action thinks about itself as having two sides, two halves of the same whole: first responders and expert scientists. And, as they move forward, their work is always about this co-development, one side learning from the other, dynamically.

So, what do those survivors of immense mortality need, before any single aircraft bearing forensic experts finds somewhere safe to land, or the army arrives, or whoever else from far away, probably days later? HFA starts with what they already have – those most basic of human instincts, to recover, identify and bury the dead – and gives them a structure from which to do that. So the survivors do what they already do, but they think about it slightly differently. They will not only be burying the dead, but also managing human remains correctly, so that, if future identification is to be enabled, key information is preserved and kept accessible, whether it comes in the form of digital photographs on mobile phones, or DNA in hair and bones. To do this, the HFA, in conjunction with the ICRC, created a how-to book, or, as it is technically known, a field manual: *Management of Dead Bodies after Disasters: A Field Manual for First Responders*. Remembering what the *A* is for, in HFA, the field manual is for use on the battlefield, or at the site of the catastrophe under whose ruins can be found those who are missing, where those who search for them also seek guidance as they do so. The field manual is available in hard copy (you can write away for them, to Geneva), or as a downloadable PDF that's not too cumbersome to print out (sixty-five pages, including all the appendices and forms). It has a cover illustration: fallen autumn leaves lying on a just-discernible background photograph of wreckage from the tsunami of 2004.[248]

The field manual is practical and honest, with no elaborate introductions, extra texts or non-essential words. It simply says, 'Immediately after a disaster there is little time to read guidelines, so this manual dedicates one chapter to each key task.' Because its authors have stood for the dead for all their professional lives, they have a very particular authority in expressing the complexities that can arise for the inexperienced. The need to be clear about what they are seeing is prime, so:

> Throughout the manual, the terms 'dead bodies', 'the deceased', or 'the dead' are used, instead of the more respectful and techni-cally correct term 'human remains', because the former are less ambiguous for readers. The term 'body part' is used to refer to tissue that is recognizably human but is less than the whole body; body parts are treated in the same manner as the whole body.

Like all good field manuals, it hopes to provide guidance for those planning for disasters before they happen, to give an indication of what might be needed most and in greatest volume (body bags, phone-charging capability and land). But that's hope; the manual is primarily intended to be used by first responders who have had no preparation, no training, and have simply begun to work, with enough battery on their phones to have downloaded it. It tells them, in straightforward language, what they are there for, and that, if they can do as much as possible, the forensic scientists that come after them will do the rest. The field manual reminds them that the priority will always be the rescue and care of survivors, but after that is taken care of, it is up to them to stand firm.

The field manual explains how handling a dead body is more difficult than everyone thinks. Two adults will generally be required to lift a single adult dead body (the manual doesn't say if only one is required for a child). It directs that the body should be lifted from the side (not end to end), with one person supporting the head and pelvic area, and one supporting the upper back and lower thigh. Then, supported in this way, bodies should be moved feet first, and put in a body bag at point of recovery. Body bags are part of the comprehensive list of essential kit to be assembled, coming under the category of something that 'ideally happens before disaster strikes', but always with the recognition that it is likely this may not have happened. The list is long, but the essentials are few (and starred ★ on the list). Other starred items are: plastic aprons, gloves, disinfectant soap, first aid kits, smaller plastic bags with closures, cable ties, waterproof labels (preferably sturdy), indelible markers or other pens, a camera (with the biggest memory and chargeable battery possible), and annex 1 and 2 downloaded from the field manual (Dead Body Data Form and Missing Persons Form).

When the body has been moved and placed into a body bag, before it is closed, it is better for everyone if the first responder makes a visual record. This is a significant change from previous practice. The forensic teams that went to Thailand had very clear, firm Interpol disaster-victim identification instructions about visual identification (looking at someone's face, either in a photograph or in real death) being ineffective, usually because of the ravages of catastrophe, time and heat. So, throughout their work, they operated on the principle that the best way to confirm a person's identity is with fingerprint, dental or DNA evidence. Humanitarian Forensic Action knows that, in situations of immense mortality, the best way is incompatible with what is possible. Visual evidence is usually all there will ever be of who it is who has died, and it can only be generated by the first responder. So, much of the field manual is taken up with how to do that.

The writers of the manual know that people doing this work won't have much time for filling in forms, so for each body, there should be a single sheet printed out, and a code generated, as many of us generate our computer passwords: letters and numbers, clear and memorable, not much information, but just enough. Three pieces of information are required to complete the form and generate the code. Firstly, the name of the place where the body was found – first responders are much better placed to work this out, because they know where they are, even if where they are is in ruins. Secondly, who is filling out the form – a number or reference for the team doing the first responding. Thirdly, a number for the body – so, if it's the thirty-fifth body they have retrieved that day, No. 35. Where, by whom, and what number = a unique code. Then it's written on two of the sturdy paper labels, and one is attached to the body itself (that's what the cable ties are for).

Next comes the visual image. First responders are usually there in time to take a high-quality photograph of the dead body, before the effects of time and heat set in (as the manual puts it, 'Sooner is better for photographing the dead'). If the first responder can photograph and label the dead as their first response, it can mean the difference between identification and the eternity of being missing, but it also means making decisions about what to photograph. People who have died as the result of head injury may be facially unrecognizable. First responders might need to clean the faces of the dead, tidy back their hair, or find other distinguishing features that can be used later on – jewellery, tattoos, clothing, or even littler things, like if their ears are pierced. They will need to become familiar with how it feels to touch and move the dead human, but that never takes very long. The manual contains sample photographs (and emphasizes that it was a live volunteer who was used as a model). Their example shows a young woman, with pierced ears, long hair and a distinctive wrist tattoo. A basic ruler has been placed by her head, for scale, and the coded paper label (place, team, first body recovered that day) is clearly readable. It is the art and practice of the possible.

And even though the ideal next step would be to keep the body cool, there is nowhere on Earth that has enough refrigeration to do this when the mortality is immense. And no dry ice, even if it seems like a good, quick solution (and they often have it in hotels) – another lesson from Thailand. Dry ice is difficult to handle and causes burns. When it melts, its run-off is toxic and polluting, and difficult to dispose of. Temporary burial is the next best option, because the temperature of the earth is always cooler than its surface. So the teams dig, as they did at Solferino, as much land as there is for long trenches, a metre and a half deep, and at least 200 metres from a water source. Once bodies have been wrapped and labelled, they can be laid in the trench – as they were at the Battle of the Somme – facing a particular direction, if faith and cultural traditions are to be respected, and then covered with a layer of earth at least ninety centimetres thick, to prevent scavenging.

Then, do it again: recover, photograph, code, wrap, bury and repeat. The field manual reminds teams to ensure someone is collecting the photographs at the end of the day and uploading them to a databank (and backing up as they go). If a rescue team is trying to find the living, those dealing with the dead should get out of their way. Any liaison with local communities should happen a little way out from where the teams are doing their work, because the sight of burial trenches is horrifying. First responders will become the liaison point for all the organizations that are coming to help, from local authorities to national militaries. The field manual asks that, as they do all this, they should seek to do it with dignity – try not to make burial look like tipping or construction work. Temporary graves should be part of the process of dignifying the dead, as well as identifying them. A temporary grave and a mass grave is not the same thing, and being clear about that will help communities recover.

Liaising with local communities will be a significant feature of the work, because first responders will quickly be identified as the people to go to when someone hasn't come home. That's why the other essential form to download and keep copies of is the missing persons form, so the first responder can keep track of everyone reported to them, without having to hold the details in their head. The field manual also asks first responders to take care of themselves.

It reminds them that what they are doing is the hardest work in the world, and not just because bodies are heavy and difficult to move. It is important that they should not put themselves at risk, because another casualty makes everything worse – one more body to recover and one less experienced first responder to do it. The field manual urges teamwork, and that members of the team should support each other and debrief at the end of the day. And if they have a question or are overwhelmed, they can read the field manual's short chapters on clearly discernible topics to find the answers. Technical information and confidence is delivered in sixty-five pages.

While I was writing this book, I was coordinator on another, more conventional field manual, which was created to support first responders to a particular group of survivors: the *Paediatric Blast Injury Field Manual. Management of Dead Bodies after Disasters: A Field Manual for First Responders* was our guide text. From it, we learned to keep the language simple, to make the important points clearly and simply, in the right order, and, above all, to always remember the people for whom we were writing. We didn't have such a meaningful cover (ours just says *Paediatric Blast Injury Field Manual* and a list of contents), but we thought hard about every single stage of recovery and the people in the field who might be handling a badly injured child for the first time (which takes a very long time to get used to).[249]

Just like the editors of *Management of Dead Bodies after Disasters*, we thought hard about what a first responder actually is, and how we could support them. For us, first responders can be bystanders, paramedics, surgeons who don't normally do paediatrics in an emergency medical facility full of children, nurses in 'critical care' wards, which are simply rooms apart from the operating theatre, in a building that may be under fire. But above all, they are local, and present, so their patient doesn't have to wait for someone else to arrive from a long way away. And because of the *Management of Dead Bodies* field manual, we included a section on what is medically termed 'futility'. Futility is when medical staff reach a point where they realize that no care will deliver the desired positive outcomes and that their patient will die, no matter what they do, and so they stop doing anything but managing pain and ensuring comfort. Futility means that, somehow, the last Horseman has entered the room. Futility is something everyone treating paediatric blast injury dreads, because children die differently from adults – they can survive extraordinarily high strain injuries, but then suddenly fall away, and we simply don't know why. Treating children is hard, deciding to stop treating them is even harder, so our manual includes a section that contains the futility decision-making quadrant, which helps medics structure their thinking about the line between the life of a child and its death. This is information they may already know, but in the turmoil of paediatric emergencies, they can't access because something in their brain won't let them. The material on futility is not a hasty page bolted on at the end, something easily passed over, because everyone would prefer not to think about it; it's facing the Horseman full on, and holding the line, so that others who might be faltering can be restored. Technical information is support, support is confidence, and confidence means that teams doing the hardest work in the world, among the living or the dead, can keep going.

In the years since its original publication, the *Management of Dead Bodies* field manual has been translated into eight languages and has been in use all over the world, by first responders and those doing disaster planning. It has also been updated, in its print and online versions. This is essential and life-saving. There's a lot of fancy talk about keeping things that go online updated, but it's rarely done. Not so with the *Management of Dead Bodies* field manual, which is a work in progress and frank about it, and it hits its own deadlines. One of the things it used to say, because it's one of the inhibitors to first response, is that the risk to first responders and to the public generally of infectious disease spreading from dead bodies is very low. Then, in 2013, the world experienced its worst Ebola outbreak (see Pestilence, above), and the *Management of Dead Bodies* field manual was rapidly updated.

Ebola is a Group 4 pathogen, which means isolation for the living and the dead, and full-body protection for those handling anyone who's been infected. Group 4 pathogens are very easily transmitted, and can live on the dead for a number of days. And this is a problem, because in many societies around the world, touching the dying, holding their hand as they slip away, is encouraged as part of the grief process. We are yet to fully understand the consequences of not being able to physically say goodbye to our loved ones who have died of COVID in hospitals, entirely isolated from us. The virus has forced a sea change in some of our longest- and hardest-held traditions and expectations of how we manage death.

All of this was foreseen in the 2013 Ebola epidemic. In the early weeks of an Ebola outbreak, when it was mistaken for the effects of other non-infectious diseases, such as malaria or sepsis, funerals were structured around washing, touching and kissing the body of the person who had died, and as the forensic humanitarians put it, in the days when very few people knew what PPE stood for, the mourners were 'obviously without personal protective equipment'.[250] One funeral in Guinea, in 2014, passed the Ebola virus on to eighteen attendees, who in turn passed it to another sixty-seven in their family circles. And while this rate of transmission is frightening, we should note that we also understand it very clearly and precisely, and that it is this ability to trace contact by local medical authorities, to understand place and time of infection, that went on to make the vaccination process so effective.

Back while the WHO leadership was still dithering in 2014, there were pockets of expertise developing on the ground, particularly in Liberia, where a system of dead-body management evolved that would become the model for good, life-saving practice in an infectious disease epidemic. The Liberian government understood that management of the dead was a key factor in keeping people safe from the virus. They knew the Liberian Red Cross had previous experience working with those killed in armed conflict in the region, and they asked them to adapt their skills. The Liberian Red Cross asked the International Committee of the Red Cross, who by then considered humanitarian forensics to be a key component of their organization, to work with them to manage the growing mortality from the Ebola virus. Together, they created four dead-body collection teams that were responsible for the collection, transport and disposal of dead bodies in the capital, Monrovia. They were joined by volunteers – first responders – who were prepared for the neces-

sity and attention to detail that the work would require. As well as
the four teams, there were eleven vehicles. Drivers didn't get out
of their cabs, so didn't have to wear personal protective equipment,
which meant they could see their way more clearly – and perhaps a
vehicle being driven by a visible human was less frightening to the
pedestrians watching from the roadsides. One of the vehicles carried
the bodies, and the other the body-recovery team. Body-recovery
teams were composed of a team leader, a scout, the team member
with spraying equipment and, hopefully, three to four volunteers to
do the wrapping and carrying. They would drive to where a death
had been reported, put on their personal protective equipment and
find their way to the dead body.

The system they developed for managing each dead body was
carefully rehearsed and carried out. It is still in use in Ebola
outbreaks today. The sprayer went inside the property first, and
sprayed the room and the body. Then the body was placed in an
open body bag and sprayed again, including all around the interior
of the bag, and then the exterior, after it was closed. Ebola is easy
to kill with disinfectant, but as the actual danger diminished, the
fear engendered by teams in PPE carrying body bags grew. We'd
all grown wary of the sight, by the end of 2020. Each Liberian
team could collect between five and ten bodies per day, but always
in an atmosphere of tension, always against a background of fear,
and sometimes anger from the local community that the death
had occurred, that Ebola was still unvanquished, that local norms
and rites were not being respected. In PPE – Ebola armour – it
was difficult to communicate with the care that these encounters

needed, so sometimes the police came along as well, to manage the tension, and, more often than not, to hold people back while the team did their work. When the vehicles were full, they drove to the crematorium, outside the city, which could cope with a capacity of fifty bodies a day. Carpentry offcuts were used for fuel in the incinerator, and it took at least six hours to accomplish the task of burning the bodies to ashes.

As the dead-body collection teams went about their work, the forensic humanitarians paid close and careful attention. They saw that the teams did extraordinary work, hampered by delays in collection and pressure on the crematoriums because of government insistence on all the dead, from whatever disease cause, being burned. And they saw that personal protective equipment worked, so all the rigmarole of getting it on and seeing through it and trying to be steady was worth it. At the end of every day, team members were sprayed one final time, before taking off their PPE and adding it to the pile for incineration, and then they went home. Discipline was consistent, and not one member of the dead-body collection teams caught Ebola. But their protection only went so far. For these local teams, there was no psychosocial support, no decompression, no debriefing, just a quick spray of disinfectant. The forensic humanitarians noted that first responders rarely get this kind of follow-up (although it's standard among trained forensic experts, wherever they are in the world) and that they should. When they asked later, local team members said that, in particular, they had felt stigmatization because of their work, and dealing with so many grieving families was just so hard, and they slept badly because of it all. Being able to tell someone about it, and to pass on what they had learned that day, the first responders felt, would have been a good thing to do.

There were other lessons the forensic humanitarians learned. Resolution is more difficult when bodies have been incinerated rather than buried. When that was the case, responders should find some way of preserving some of the ashes from each burn, and labelling them, so they could be put in a suitable memorial once the disaster was over.[251] Their main learning was that, ten years after the first edition of the *Management of Dead Bodies* field manual, 'scientific and technical developments in the field suggested an update was necessary'. Ebola, in 2013, made it essential. Today's field manual has a section on dealing with the bodies of persons who have died from an epidemic of infectious disease, and unlike the rest of the manual, which can be used by the untrained – as long as they have pens, labels and plastic sheeting – this section is *not* for untrained first responders, very specifically. Accordingly, the list of essential kit for those handling people killed by a Group 4 pathogen is much longer, and begins with training, and then includes the personal protective equipment that we became so familiar with in 2020. Face shields and goggles, fluid-resistant non-collapsible surgical facemasks, double nitrile gloves (nitrile materials are stronger than latex, and a double glove is 90 per cent better than a single one, no matter how thick) with long cuffs. And, ideally, waterproof single-use aprons that can be torn off with double nitrile gloved hands and burned, and gum boots (that can be thoroughly washed), and a head cover. And self-discipline, the life-saving kind shown in Monrovia, 'to follow the procedures correctly and without exception'. And once again, the importance of doing the paperwork is stressed, and the need to create a marker to show where remains or the ashes of remains lie, so that families may one day go there in the hope of finding resolution, and in the meantime, they will know that time and care was taken with their departed.

In 2020, the *Management of Dead Bodies* field manual was not updated, but the technical guidance it gives to first responders and those planning for the management of the dead outside medical facilities remains correct and necessary, in a time when everyone knows what PPE stands for. The forensic unit at the ICRC did compile an article which reiterated the field manual's key points, though, and published it in the leading international forensic-science journal. Their primary concern was to emphasize that the COVID-19 pandemic was no excuse not to ensure dignified and professional management of each deceased individual whose death contributed to the statistics that so horrified the world every time they turned on the nightly news briefings. Perhaps the authors of the article had seen the images of rushed burial early in the pandemic, because one point in particular was emphasized (and it's their bold text, not mine): 'Mass graves are **highly discouraged**. They are often a demonstration of poor planning by authorities, [and] show a disregard for the wishes, cultural/religious rites of families and communities. Single graves are respectful and dignified, they promote the traceability of human remains.'[252]

Off the coast of Aceh, as the new year of 2005 dawns, the pale rider waits for the other Horsemen to join him. From what he can see of the remains of the coast, it promises rich pickings – richer if they work together.

After the water had moved on, the land settled in contours that could be mapped once more, although it had permanently subsided by several metres, and was poisoned by seawater and toxins. Lights were still low, because few utilities remained. Eighty per cent of the water supply and most of the sewage lines were broken, and the smashing of the rest of the district's communication infrastructure meant their restoration would be slow. As an absolute priority, the humanitarian agencies had set up camps for the hundreds of thousands of displaced families who had come into their care. Hourly deliveries of huge tanks of clean water were made, and every day there were queues of people waiting with empty plastic bottles to collect their allocation for drinking, cooking and washing. There had been cholera in Aceh two years earlier, and acute diarrhoea among its children, measurable as serious since 2001.[253] There hadn't been much malnutrition to speak of before the tsunami, but afterwards, brackish standing water pools all over the abandoned land were the ideal breeding ground for waterborne diseases and insects, as was any contaminated drinking water, and the degradation of digestive and immune systems would surely follow, and then wasting and stunting.

But the other Horsemen never came, even though the world had cracked open along a 1,300-kilometre gap – plenty of room for all of them, and this was, after all, how they originally rode

out on to the earth.* A line of national and international humanitarian resources had been drawn up ahead of them. The WHO
coordinated teams that fogged insecticides over the stagnant water,
while an entirely new system of water pipelines replaced old and
destroyed versions.[254] A modern sewage system was installed and
connected throughout the province. The new, safe system threaded
its way into the refugee camps and tented cities where the citizens
and their families were now living, and medics gave talks and put
up posters about the dangers of waterborne diseases. Proper pipes,
public awareness and public health meant that diarrhoea rates
actually fell after the tsunami event, and the rates have stayed low
ever since. And there was no cholera at all. There was one small
outbreak of a rotavirus in a refugee camp in 2007, but it was easily
contained and treated – no wasting, no stunting. New systems of
water, sewage and disease surveillance closed gaps that had been
open for decades.

And there was nothing, it turned out, for War either, even though
the blood-red horse was already very familiar with the soft hills,
dunes, cities and villages of Aceh. There had been civil war between
the local separatist movement and the national government since
1976.[255] It was proper violent war, with thousands of deaths, and
the constant threat of violence was part of everyday life. It stemmed
from older colonial struggles from the time when the region was
called Java, and was complicated by religious, social and economic

---

* Revelation 6:1: 'And I saw when the Lamb opened one of the seals, and I heard,
as it were the noise of thunder, one of the four beasts saying, Come and see.'

entanglements. People had moved from the cities to get out of the way of the fighting, pushed to the coasts to scrape new lives and live-lihoods where the land met the sea. There had been many attempts to negotiate an end to the conflict, all ending in failure. In 2003, the government declared a state of emergency in the province to control the never-ending cycle of violence and displacement. The state of emergency was why so many Indonesian troops were in Aceh when the tsunami struck, and how they were able to assist the process of burial that otherwise would have taken so many more weeks and months to complete (and why we know the numbers on the grim little graph).

And whatever the state of Aceh may have been on 25 December 2004, it was clear by nightfall on 26 December that things were going to have to change. Relief and reconstruction would require, above all, peace. So, as the engineers and road-builders and human-itarians went in, the warring sides sat down with Finnish mediators in Helsinki to build something equally important. By August 2005, they had signed a peace treaty ending thirty years of war. There was an immediate ceasefire.[256] Weapons were handed in (any working device with a steel chamber and steel barrel constituted a weapon, including guns, rifles, grenade launchers and shoulder-fired mis-sile launchers). There was an amnesty for separatist fighters and a release of prisoners. Half the military and police forces in Aceh – those not needed for tsunami recovery duties – were recalled. Aceh achieved the separate status it had longed for, together with its own flag, crest and anthem. Aceh-based parties were able to participate in politics. It got to keep most of the money from the region's mineral reserves. In agreement with the national government, sharia law, long preferred by the Muslim majority in Aceh, replaced secular law. And in came the paraphernalia of peacekeeping to hold the new line: international monitors, truth and reconciliation commissions, humanitarian liaison offices. There were safe spaces and ways of reporting treaty violations, promises being seen to be quickly kept. The local population was kept up to date with the process of peace, and why, this time, it was different (not that they needed reminding). In six months, faced with immense mortality, peace became possible.

Just as in Mosul, as soon as things were safe, a team went into Aceh to survey the consequences of the catastrophe for the individuals, households and communities they found there. They had a sense of what they were looking for, and an equally strong sense of what had disappeared. In Aceh, nine months before the tsunami, there had been a population census, conducted by Statistics Indonesia, that covered 800,000 households chosen to represent the district level of each province. A census can be a difficult thing to undertake, especially in a country as geographically complicated as Indonesia, with remote districts and villages, and entire provinces engaged in civil wars. But the government has considerable experience in doing them, and they are overseen by international statistical authorities, several of which had been involved with Statistics Indonesia for decades.

The Study of the Tsunami Aftermath and Recovery (STAR, from now on) was a collaboration of Statistics Indonesia, Survey-METER (Indonesia), several US universities specializing in population studies and public health, and the World Bank. STAR's work began by analysing the actual site of such immense mortality, and the descriptor is theirs. Because these were places where lives and landscapes were lived and destroyed inseparably, STAR analysed physical and geographic destruction as well as human. Those photographs we all clicked on which showed the before and after coastlines were taken by the team. They were the ones who asked for the images of light and then darkness on the first evening after the wave struck, from the remote sensor arrays on satellites overhead. They were the first to quantify the amount of newly created bare earth in Aceh (either from scouring or salinated sediment deposition). They asked community leaders for their assessment of the damage and took their own GPS measurements.

And then they went to look for the survivors who were still there, living on the land. The aim of the study was to find as many households as possible that had been counted in the previous census, to interview everyone aged eleven or over, and ask them about any younger children. They aimed for 585 study sites, in three kinds of district: those directly affected by the tsunami, those not directly affected, and those not affected at all, as a control group. It took until May 2005 for the tracker teams to identify and contact relevant cases, but they managed it, somehow, in all that debris. By the time the work began, they had 28,372 respondents from 7,000 households, who sat quietly and answered the questions, pausing for the researchers to tick the boxes on their forms. Interviewing all of them for the first time took about a year.

Everything we know and use today to understand who lived and who died in the tsunami comes from the work of STAR.

This is aftermath analytics, done not just as figures, but rigorously, and accounting for temporal or spatial variation in the surveillance sensitivity; STAR demographers incorporated compassion as an exceptional emergency measure, without which the true picture of the courage of the people of Aceh would never have been known. They listened to the stories of survivors, and learned that, despite the pace and scale of the wave, 'the picture that emerges is not one in which household members panicked blindly but rather one of families in which stronger members sought to help those they could – in some cases successfully, in others not.'[257]

Of those who survived, who were tracked to where they'd fled and sought shelter, only 1 per cent decided not to participate in the STAR survey when its staff asked them to consider it. Or STAR1, as that survey is now known. Because, having achieved what no one else has ever managed, STAR investigators kept going, answering the question that is at the heart of what makes us living humans: what happens when we do not die? There have been five follow-up studies, with the last (and ten-year follow-up) conducted in 2014 – STAR6. The structure of the study was able to incorporate new members – children who grew into adults, new wives and families. Study subjects stayed loyal to STAR. Drop-off rate for participation was very low – if people moved out of tents, out of refugee camps, into their own homes once again, they told the STAR coordinators. STAR itself says that it is the strongest large-scale longitudinal study ever done to measure population-level response to a disaster. It is exactly right, but it's also more than that.

The STAR studies are acts of compassion, consideration and hope, and data analysis, all seriously and patiently done. Like all the studies in this book (especially those 3,000 extraordinary neonates and their families who participated in the sepsis study), they provide a reminder to us of what is possible and necessary if we are prepared to take the time that truth and understanding require. After the tsunami, many studies rushed to conclude that it was the poor and displaced that died at Aceh. STAR's findings cohered with those of the seismologists: socio-economic factors played no role in whether or not someone died. No one gets away in fifteen minutes. STAR2 was watching as the first babies were born and it noted that the ones who were in utero at the time of the tsunami were stunted in their first thousand days, but they caught up. STAR may need to coordinate with the nutrition scientists about what constitutes catch-up, but their numbers tell us that sudden stressful occurrences can be compensated for, and that understanding this mechanism may be helpful with other forms of catch-up, and we have a good, well-populated data set in which to start looking. STAR work has looked at whether this kind of extreme stress has an effect on an individual's long-term physiology. We tend to think it might, but because we can't do very long studies (or we haven't tried hard enough), we don't know. STAR2 (2006) incorporated cardiometabolic biomarker monitoring of 5,000 of their study participants, specifically by looking at diabetes rates. It found that there was no difference in the rates of diabetes onset between the communities that were severely damaged and those that were not damaged at all.[258] The stress, in all its horror, went away, with no long-term physiological effects. It's that kind of data that makes Death splash back, out of sight from the coast of Aceh. There was survival and life beyond survival, and it was no less or more healthy than anywhere else in the world.

STAR was watching as, slowly, villages and families were rebuilt amid the silt and scouring, as something like $7 billion was spent restoring the province.[259] People wanted to come home – people always want to come home, even when the scouring is by explosives and the earth is hidden under rubble – and by STAR4, communities were growing from in-migration. Immense mortality is usually followed by an increase in fertility, and so it was in Aceh. STAR saw that the group of survivors who paid the highest price were those who were teenagers when the tsunami struck, and had to leave school and go to work to support the remnants of their families or communities. Their findings supported other conclusions that adolescents always have it hard, when times are hard, and that we need to pay attention to this, wherever or for whatever reason the hard times occur.

As well as looking at long-term physiological effects, STAR incorporated mental health questions into their survey. They did it by asking participants to think of a six-step ladder, with the bottom rung meaning they were feeling at their lowest. In STAR1, they found very high rates of PTSD in communities marked as severely affected by the tsunami – many people crowded on to the lowest rung of the ladder, clinging on for dear life. But as each study progressed, the participants moved upwards, rung by rung. And their satellite images confirmed what their questionnaires concluded. Roads once again wove their way back into villages and towns, fields and boundaries were once again discernible, and the lights went back on. There is resilience – post-traumatic growth – in environments with new schools, new water systems – especially water. If attacks on utilities are effectively attacks on medical facilities, then each time a water-treatment facility opens and gets going, and there is no waterborne disease, it's as good as rebuilding the health infrastructure – two for the price of one. The Multi-Donor Fund that handled the reconstruction financing run by the World Bank was rightly very keen on being able to do things like this.

Much of the rebuilding of Aceh was done by 2008, and that, in itself, was a problem, because the humanitarian spend was huge (the 'reconstruction dividend'), and skewed the economic growth and employment figures. That's something that often happens – at Mosul, the non-traditional coalition paid above local average wages, which made things difficult for traditional humanitarians who didn't. In Aceh, after the reconstruction, trade and transport were no longer needed, and the clearing of tsunami debris was finished, so the economy shrank. The lights flickered because some of the newly built power facilities weren't always reliable, and investors were worried about local crime rates, which meant businesses were paying for either security or protection. And the World Bank noted that many of the big organizations who had done the work of the reconstruction hadn't really thought about their exit strategy – 'smooth project closure'. So they kept working, for a little longer, to make sure that jobs transferred out, that local government could take over in a way that didn't marginalize or exclude communities, or aggravate ethnic tensions, and this extension phase was effective.[260] The participants in the STAR5 survey, begun in 2009, had kept on climbing the ladder.

'Smooth project closure' helped hold the line in Aceh, because it held the peace. In 2010, the original architects of the peace treaty created a follow-up project to assess progress and resilience. It reported in 2012, and felt confident enough in what it found to describe the findings as a 'Final Report'. Most web-based material on the peace process in Aceh has been archived, although it's difficult to say that the job has been completely done (or, as the outbreak analyst would say, 'give a good confident end of outbreak declaration'), because there remain concerns about truth and reconciliation, and whether peace has brought all the justice there should be.[261] Sharia law has been extended and consolidated, and this has led to profound concerns about the criminalization of aspects of LGBT life and community and the resumption of corporal punishment in public for a broad and puzzling range of what most other countries in the world would not recognize as offences.[262] The people of Aceh will have to resolve these issues, but now they have the political and social means, and it's their work to do, not that of any other government or humanitarian agency.

Along its new coastline, the sea still rolls in and out, as and where it should. The government has done the hard work on disaster risk reduction – with flood reduction measures, and building stronger, taller houses. It connected up to a tsunami early-warning system in the Indian Ocean, built after 2004 and coordinated by UNESCO (who are also at the heart of the reconstruction of Mosul, after the horror of its destruction, although an early-warning system for peril approaching the world's oldest city is not their mandate) – although everyone recognizes that early warnings are still not much help for island communities so close to active fault lines, what *National Geographic* magazine has called 'an unforgiving margin between life and death'.[263] There are sirens and drills, and vertical evacuation centres, built strongly, so people can climb their way above the water and stay there until the next wave has passed over. There have been other seismic events, much smaller and altogether less impactful; the public response didn't go as well as had been hoped for, and the evacuation centres were locked and no one knew where the key was, but the problems weren't anything that wasn't readily fixable, with some practice. Death can too easily find his way to the Sumatra–Andaman fault line, without any help from humankind, but there is still no room for the rest of his cohort.

2012 was a year of resolution in Aceh, and of rigorous surveillance to ensure high confidence in the declaration of the end of the catastrophe (outbreak analytic scientists would approve). There was a short final report from the stewards of the peace process, and a longer report and conference from the World Bank and the Multi-Donor Fund. The STAR6 study, completed in 2014, is the last demographic survey to date. As both interviewer and interviewee knew the process and each other well by then, it focused on updating information on education, work, marriage, new families, new kinship networks; hopes, dreams and expectations becoming more familiar. All the reports, taken together, show the great rolling force of resilient peace – peace that everyone has got used to living in, including the generation growing up today, who know nothing else and have only ever heard about the tsunami, because almost all the signs of its destruction are gone.

As the pale rider splashes back across the oceans to find the rest of his company, he sees that, in all the parts of the line held against him, work is being consistently consolidated. It turns out that we are already building the second age of humanitarianism, starting with the radical reordering of one of Dunant's first principles. Working for the dead is really working for the living at the same time. No one can do one without, in some way, doing the other. It may have taken a while to cohere around that single point, but today the International Committee of the Red Cross sees Humanitarian Forensic Action as a key component of its portfolio. It's official. They said it themselves, in March 2020: 'The ICRC acquired forensic capability in the early 2000s to support its humanitarian operations around the world, including for ensuring the proper and dignified management, documentation and identification of the dead.'[264]

There are ninety forensic specialists working for the ICRC now, overseen and advised by the originators of the concept of Humanitarian Forensic Action. Though no one is taking anything for granted; capability acquired can always be sidelined. So, the ICRC forensics unit keeps pace with the science across all the fields around the world that could possibly be relevant to their practice, and they've built one of the most extraordinary networks of multidisciplinary experts anywhere on our planet today. At the same time, they keep the balance between cutting-edge science and the extreme demands of first response. They are still not necessarily looking for the best, but are focusing on what's possible – what capabilities can be readily moved to the front of the line, so the humans that stand there for the dead can begin work right away.

Whatever is necessary to secure their community of practice as something sustainable, humanitarian forensic scientists are ready to do (and for them, it's always intensively sustainable). They are able to summarize the current state of haemogenetics, as well as cite the exact detail of the sections on humanity after life from the articles of international humanitarian law. They can assess how long a human being may have been held in confinement, or what kind of torture they have endured. Increasingly, their work is to establish identities for the living missing: for children, or the deeply traumatized, or elderly people in refugee camps or battleground cities, who no longer know how old they are, or where they have come from, or who they once were. In March 2020, following a request by governments and other relevant stakeholders, the ICRC issued the detailed 'General Guidance for the Management of the Dead Related to COVID-19'. There was no one else for governments and stakeholders to ask, and no one better. We've achieved so much for the second age of humanitarianism by starting from its very hardest point. Surely, hopefully, we can do the rest – as we should, after Mosul. And if death is not the end of the line, then there is no end of the line, there are no passing places, and no gaps. The Horsemen can keep trying to find new paths through, but they'll never succeed, because no matter how hard the ground or dark the storm clouds, there will always be extraordinary people standing in their way.

Author's Note

At the end of the conversations I had for this book, everyone told me something simple and essential. I don't mean that in the metaphorical sense. They actually told me to write down that there are fundamental truths in their work, as they understand them, beyond the science they do every day. From my notes, here they are.

Good communication is the essence of stewardship.

Good governance is the only possible infrastructure on which to build a healthcare system.

The malnutrition of children is, more than anything else, about the waste of human potential.

Good children's healthcare is founded on nurturing. If a child is nurtured, everything else will follow.

This is the simple and essential truth at the heart of my work: there are more people working in our world for good than any other kind. When I started to follow the line, I don't think I ever expected to find either the strength or the numbers working there. It isn't just that there are people in the way of the Horsemen, it's that there are so very many of them, working alongside each other, on behalf of the rest of us. We need to get back into the habit of looking for them, staying with them, understanding what it is they are doing. Perhaps – now I come to think about it – that's why the Horsemen have tracked us into our own time. So that, when we remember ancient danger, we can also envisage new hope.

Emily Mayhew
Imperial College London, 2021

Endnotes

Introduction

1   Thank you to Professor Olivette Otele, who recently described her
    own historian-activism in a lecture at the Chelsea History Festival,
    25 September 2020.

PART ONE: WAR

2   Thomas Davies, *NGOs: A New History of Transnational Civil Society*
    (London: Hurst & Co. 2013), p. 37.
3   Caroline Moorhead, *Dunant's Dream* (London: HarperCollins,
    1998), pp. 1–22.
4   Henri Dunant, *A Memory of Solferino* (Geneva: ICRC, 1939, 1959),
    PDF, translated, p. 127.
5   See Davies, *NGOs*.
6   Christine Okrent, Peter Maurer, speeches at the November 2019
    Paris Peace Forum opening session, https://parispeaceforum.org/
    program-2019.

7   Paul Wise, Paul Spiegel et al., *The Mosul Trauma Response: A Case Study* (Baltimore, MD: Johns Hopkins Center for Humanitarian Health, 2018), p. 21.

8   J. Bonomi, *Nineveh and its Palaces* (London: Bohn, 1857), p. 4.

9   Peter Frankopan, *The Silk Roads* (London: Bloomsbury, 2015), p. 70.

10   Robert Hillenbrand, *Islamic Art and Architecture* (London: Thames & Hudson, 1999), p. 419.

11   Martin Frishman and Hasan-Uddin Khan (eds.), *The Mosque* (London: Thames & Hudson, 2002).

12   Ibid, p. 24.

13   See entry for Ibn al-Athir, Abu al-Hasan Ali Izz al-Din in *The Oxford Dictionary of Islamic Studies*. Al-Athir was one of three brothers who travelled widely and wrote works of historical and linguistic scholarship.

14   See *The Travels of Ibn Jubayr: A Medieval Journey from Cordoba to Jerusalem* (London: IB Tauris, 2019), p. 263.

15   See Miroslav Melčák and Ondrej Beránek, 'ISIS's Destruction of Mosul's Historical Monuments: Between Media Spectacle and Religious Doctrine', in *International Journal of Islamic Architecture*, Vol. 6, No. 2, July 2017.

16   For work on the sharing of sacred spaces in Muslim cities, see Stephennie Mulder, *The Shrines of the 'Alids in Medieval Syria: Sunnis, Shi'is and the Architecture of Coexistence* (Edinburgh: Edinburgh University Press, 2014).

17   Frishman and Khan (eds), *The Mosque*, p. 58.

18   For details of these integrated acts of thought and worship, see H. U. Khan et al. (eds), *International Journal of Islamic Architecture*, Vol.1.

19   John Philip Newman, *Thrones and Palaces of Babylon and Nineveh* (London: Hardpress Publishing, 2012), p. 286.

20 Yakou Malko, 'At the Mercy of the Elements: Cultural Preservation of Ancient Sites in Mosul (Nineveh Province)', in *International Journal of Contemporary Iraqi Studies*, Vol. 7, No. 2, June 2013.

21 'Cinemas for Mosul: A Call for the International Community', The Mosul Eye, 30 June 2019.

22 Falah Al-Kubaisy, *Mosul: The Architectural Conservation in Mosul Old Town – Iraq* (2010).

23 See James Verini, *They Will Have to Die Now* (New York: W. W. Norton, 2020), which is the first work to pay proper attention to a range of these sources.

24 The Mosul Eye, posted 18 June 2014. The website has the archive of all his posts: https://mosul-eye.org/2014/06/18/230pm-1762014-mosul-what-i-have-witnessed-today-is-very-difficult-to-express-in-writing-there-are-lots-of-fabrications-and-false-news-that-have-been-spread-by-media-however-they-are-contradict.

25 Melčák and Beránek, 'ISIS's Destruction of Mosul's Historical Monuments'.

26 For a full description of the genocidal atrocities perpetrated on the Yazidis, see Nadia Murad, *The Last Girl* (London: Virago, 2018), and its accompanying documentary.

27 Valeria Cetorelli et al. 'Mortality and Kidnapping Estimates for the Yazidi Population in the Area of Mount Sinjar, Iraq, in August 2014: A Retrospective Household Survey', in *PLoS Med* Vol. 14, No. 5, May 2017.

28 See John M. Quinn, Omar F. Amouri and Pete Reed, 'Notes from a Field Hospital South of Mosul', in *Globalization and Health* Vol. 14, No. 27, 2018, p. 2.

29 Riyadh Lafta, Valeria Cetorelli and Gilbert Burnham, 'Health and Health Seeking in Mosul during ISIS Control and Liberation: Results From a 40-Cluster Household Survey', in *Disaster Medicine and Public Health Preparedness*, Vol. 13, No. 4, August 2019.

30   Mosul Eye Report, *Education in Mosul Under ISIL's Rule: Soft Resistance and Civil Disobedience*, 2015, https://mosuleye.files.wordpress.com/2015/12/mosul-eye-education-under-isil.pdf.

31   United Nations Environment Programme, *Technical Note – Environmental Issues in Areas Retaken from ISIL [ISIS] Mosul, Iraq, Rapid Scoping Mission, July–August 2017*.

32   See Stephen A. Bourque, *Au-delà des plages: La guerre des Alliés contre la France* (Paris: Passés Composés, 2019).

33   Gary Volesky and R. Noble, 'Theater Land Operations', in *Military Review*, Vol. 97, September–October 2017, p. 23.

34   Mosul Study Group, *What the Battle for Mosul Teaches the Force*, US Army publication, No. 17-24 U, September 2017.

35   Thomas D. Arnold and Nicolas Fiore, 'Five Operational Lessons from the Battle of Mosul', in *Military Review*, Vol. 99, No. 1, January–February 2019.

36   According to *The Mosul Trauma Response* (see note 7), p. 18, the figure is 90 per cent.

37   US Department of Defense, 'Weekly Islamic State of Iraq and Syria (ISIS) Cost Report through June 30, 2017', https://dod.defense.gov/OIR/Cost/.

38   *Mosul Trauma Response*, p. 11.

39   Ibid., p. 44, 'Lessons Learned and Recommendations'.

40   Ibid., p. 11.

41   See Mosul Eye posts, 18 October to 6 November 2016.

42   Arnold and Fiore, 'Five Operational Lessons from the Battle of Mosul', p. 62.

43   Quinn, Amouri and Reed, 'Notes from a Field Hospital South of Mosul', p. 3.

44   Arnold and Fiore, 'Five Operational Lessons from the Battle of Mosul', p. 65.

45   Mosul Study Group, *What the Battle for Mosul Teaches the Force*, p. 20.

46   Riyadh Lafta, Maha A. Al-Nuaimi and Gilbert Burnham, 'Injury

and Death During the ISIS Occupation of Mosul and its Liberation: Results from a 40-Cluster Household Survey', in *PLoS Med*, Vol. 15, No. 5, 15 May 2018.

47　Georgia J. Michlig et al., 'Providing Healthcare under ISIS: A Qualitative Analysis of Healthcare Worker Experiences in Mosul, Iraq between June 2014 and June 2017', in *Global Public Health*, Vol. 14, No. 10, April 2019.

48　Lafta, Al-Nuaimi and Burnham, 'Injury and Death during the ISIS Occupation of Mosul and its Liberation'.

49　Cetorelli et al., 'Mortality and Kidnapping Estimates for the Yazidi Population', pp. 7, 8, 9, etc.

50　Françoise Cloarec, *L'Âme du Savon D'Alep* (Paris: Les Éditions Noirs sur Blanc, 2013).

51　Marcia Brophy (ed.), 'An Unbearable Reality' (Save the Children, 2017).

52　Mosul Study Group, *What the Battle for Mosul Teaches the Force*, p. 21.

53　Dr Tedros Ghebreyesus, opening speech at the inaugural Global Burden of Disease forum, reported in the *Lancet*, 5 January 2019.

54　*Mosul Trauma Response*, p. 17.

55　All ICRC annual reports are downloadable from their website. See https://www.icrc.org/data/files/annual-report-2016/regions/near-and-middle-east.pdf, pp. 21–24 for references to the aftermath of Mosul.

56　Pierre Krähenbühl, 'There Are no "Good" or "Bad" civilians in Syria – We Must Help All Who Need Aid', in *Guardian*, 3 March 2013.

PART TWO: PESTILENCE

57　Patricia E. Reed et al., 'A New Approach for Monitoring Ebolavirus in Wild Great Apes', in *PLoS Neglected Tropical Diseases* Vol. 8, No. 9, September 2014, E3143, 10.1371/journal.pntd.0003143.

58   Guojie Zhang et al., 'Comparative Analysis of Bat Genomes Pro-
      vides Insight into the Evolution of Flight and Immunity', in *Science*,
      25 January 2013.

59   Denis Malvy et al., 'Ebola Virus Disease', in the *Lancet*, Vol. 393, 2
      March 2019.

60   Thank you to my editor, Jon Riley, for pointing out this comparison
      point. Derek Gatherer, 'The 2014 Ebola Virus Disease Outbreak
      in West Africa', in *Journal of General Virology*, Vol. 95, No. 8, August
      2014.

61   Anja Wolz, 'Face to Face with Ebola – An Emergency Care Center
      in Sierra Leone', in *New England Journal of Medicine*, 18 September
      2014.

62   Gustaf Drevin et al., '"For This One, Let Me Take the Risk": Why
      Surgical Staff Continued to Perform Caesarean Sections during the
      2014–2016 Ebola Epidemic in Sierra Leone', in *BMJ Global Health*
      Vol. 4, No. 4, July 2019, e001361.

63   Joanne Liu, 'MSF International President United Nations Special
      Briefing on Ebola', 2 September 2014, https://www.msf.org/msf-in-
      ternational-president-united-nations-special-briefing-ebola.

64   This process is described in Marcos Cueto, Theodore M. Brown
      and Elizabeth Fee, *The World Health Organization: A History* (Cam-
      bridge: Cambridge University Press, 2019), pp. 320–6.

65   Although this is: *Phil Trans A* covers the physical sciences; *Phil Trans
      B* covers the life sciences. The Royal Society has a range of other
      journals, but it's *Phil Trans* which has the legendary status of having
      published Isaac Newton and everyone else from then on.

66   Oliver Morgan, 'How Decision Makers Can Use Quantitative
      Approaches to Guide Outbreak Responses', in 'Modelling Infec-
      tious Disease Outbreaks in Humans, Animals and Plants: Epidemic
      Forecasting and Control' theme issue of *Phil Trans B*, Vol. 374, No.
      1776, 8 July 2019.

67 Andrew Czyzewski, 'Modelling an Unprecedented Pandemic', https://www.imperial.ac.uk/stories/coronavirus-modelling/

68 Richard Kwasnicki, Super et al., 'Facial Pressure Injuries in Health-care Workers from FFP3 masks during the COVID-19 Pandemic', in the BAPRAS journal.

69 Maxwell J. Smith et al., 'Emergency Use Authorisation for COVID-19 Vaccines: Lessons from Ebola', in the *Lancet*, 5 November 2020.

70 Yogi Berra, on the chances of his baseball team winning the 1973 National League Pennant Race; and Robin N. Thompson, Oliver W. Morgan and Katri Jalava, 'Rigorous Surveillance is Necessary for High Confidence in End-of-Outbreak Declarations for Ebola and other Infectious Diseases', in 'Modelling Infectious Disease Outbreaks in Humans, Animals and Plants' theme issue of *Phil Trans B*, Vol. 374, No. 1776, 8 July 2019.

71 David K. Evans, Markus Goldstein and Anna Popova, 'Health-Care Worker Mortality and the Legacy of the Ebola Epidemic', in the *Lancet*, Vol. 3, No. 8, August 2015, e439; WHO press release, 'Dead and injured following attacks on Ebola responders in the Democratic Republic of the Congo', 28 November 2019.

72 David R. Wessner, 'The Origins of Viruses', *Nature Education* Vol. 3, No. 9, 2010.

73 David Moore, *Fungal Biology in the Origin and Emergence of Life* (Cambridge: Cambridge University Press, 2013), p. 3.

74 Andrew J. Surman et al., 'Environmental Control Programs the Emergence of Distinct Functional Ensembles from Unconstrained Chemical Reactions', in *PNAS* Vol. 116, No. 12, 6 March 2019.

75 Moore, *Fungal Biology*, p. 132.

76 NASA factsheet, 'Mars 2020/Perseverance' (NASA/JPL-Caltech), March 2020.

77 Jane S. Greaves et al., 'Phosphine Gas in the Cloud Decks of Venus', in *Nature Astronomy*, 14 September 2020.

78 Ulrich R. Christensen et al., 'Saturn's Magnetic Field and Dynamo', in Baines, Flasar, Krupp and Stallard (eds), *Saturn in the 21st Century* (Cambridge: Cambridge University Press, 2018), pp. 69–96.

79 Daniel Dykhuizen, 'Species Numbers in Bacteria', in *Proceedings. California Academy of Sciences*, 3 June 2005, Vol. 56 (Supp I, No. 6), p. 69.

80 Hans-Curt Flemming et al., 'Biofilms: An Emergent Form of Bacterial Life', in *Nature Reviews Microbiology*, Vol. 14, August 2016.

81 See the work and multiple publications from the Endres Lab, Imperial College London, https://www.imperial.ac.uk/people/r.endres/research.html.

82 Xiaoling Zhai et al., 'Statistics of Correlated Percolation in a Bacterial Community', in *PLoS Computational Biology*, Vol. 15, No. 12, e1007508, 2 December 2019, https://doi.org/10.1371/journal.pcbi.1007508.

83 Alexander Fleming, Nobel Lecture, 11 December 1945, p. 8, https://www.nobelprize.org/uploads/2018/06/fleming-lecture.pdf.

84 Eric Lax, *The Mould in Dr Florey's Coat* (London: Abacus, 2005).

85 George E. Shambaugh, 'History of Sulfonamides', in *Arch Otolaryngol*, Vol. 83, No. 1, January 1966.

86 Michael Stanes (ed.), *Memoirs of Edward Laidlaw Thompson, VRD, MD, FRCP* (unpublished), p. 42.

87 Justin Barr and Scott H. Podolsky, 'A National Medical Response to Crisis – The Legacy of World War II', in *New England Journal of Medicine*, 13 August 2020.

88 'Antimicrobial Resistance: Tackling a Crisis for the Health and Wealth of Nations', published by the Review on Antimicrobial Resistance, chaired by Jim O'Neill, December 2014, p. 3.

89 Nothing I came up with, unfortunately – see Alex Berezow, 'Discovered: 4th Major Mechanism for Antibiotic Resistance to Spread' on the American Council on Science and Health website, 8 September 2017.

90   Hannah Landecker, 'Antibiotic Resistance and the Biology of History', in *Body & Society*, Vol. 22, No. 4, December 2016.

91   Marc Mendelson et al., 'Antibiotic Resistance Has a Language Problem', in *Nature*, Vol. 545, 4 May 2017.

92   Dykhuizen, 'Species Numbers in Bacteria'.

93   Anton Y. Peleg, Harald Seifert and David L. Paterson, '*Acinetobacter baumannii*: Emergence of a Successful Pathogen', in *Clinical Microbiology Reviews,* July 2008, pp. 538–82.

94   In *Game of Thrones*, 'sentinel' is a title held by the second in command to the Lord of Ironrath, and, traditionally, to the head of House Forrester.

95   Sam P. Brown, Daniel M. Cornforth and Nicole Mideo, 'Evolution of Virulence in Opportunistic Pathogens: Generalism, Plasticity and Control', in *Trends in Microbiology*, Vol. 20, No. 7, July 2012, p. 336.

96   Flemming et al., 'Biofilms: An Emergent Form of Bacterial Life'.

97   Peleg, Seifert and Paterson, '*Acinetobacter baumannii*: Emergence of a Successful Pathogen', pp. 542–3. See preamble for https://www.acinetobacter2019.com.

98   Lisa L. Maragakis et al., 'An Outbreak of Multidrug-Resistant *Acinetobacter baumannii* Associated with Pulsatile Lavage Wound Treatment', in *JAMA*, Vol. 292, No. 24, pp. 3006–11, 22/29 December 2004.

99   See S. D. Henriksen, '*Moraxella, Acinetobacter* and the *Mimeae*', in *Bacteriological Reviews*, Vol. 37, No. 4, pp. 522–61.

100   Chui Yoke Chin et al., 'A High-Frequency Phenotypic Switch Links Bacterial Virulence and Environmental Survival in *Acinetobacter baumannii*', in *Nature Microbiology*, Vol. 3, No. 5, April 2018, p. 563.

101   Kovalchuk P. Valentine and Kondratiuk M. Viacheslav, 'Bacterial Flora of Combat Wounds from Eastern Ukraine and Time-Specified Changes of Bacterial Recovery during Treatment in Ukrainian

Military Hospital', in *BMC Research Notes*, Vol. 10, No. 152, 7 April 2017.

102 Mihail R. Halachev et al., 'Genomic Epidemiology of a Protracted Hospital Outbreak Caused by Multi-Drug Resistant *Acinetobacter baumannii* in Birmingham, England', in *Genome Medicine*, Vol. 6, No. 11, 2014, p. 70.

103 Peleg, Seifert and Paterson, '*Acinetobacter baumannii*: Emergence of a Successful Pathogen', in *Clinical Microbiology Reviews*, July 2008, p. 559. See also Emily Mayhew, *A Heavy Reckoning: War, Medicine and Survival in Afghanistan and Beyond* (London: Wellcome Collection, 2017), pp. 169–70.

104 https://www.walmart.com/ip/AZO-UH-DEFENSE-24CT/50274881.

105 Author's correspondence with Dr Martin Moody, urologist, Northern Devon Healthcare Trust, 10 March 2019. See also Saeed Khoshnood et al., 'Drug-Resistant Gram-Negative Uropathogens: A Review', in *Journal of Biomedicine and* Pharmacotherapy, Vol. 94, October 2017, pp. 982–94.

106 Massimo Filippini, Giuliano Masiero and Karine Moschetti, 'Socioeconomic Determinants of Regional Differences in Outpatient Antibiotic Consumption: Evidence from Switzerland', in *Health Policy* Vol. 78, No. 1, 22 August 2006, pp. 77–92; Dominik Glinz et al., 'Quality of Antibiotic Prescribing of Swiss Primary Care Physicians with High Prescription Rates: a Nationwide Survey', in *Journal of Antimicrobial Chemotherapy* Vol. 72, No. 11, 1 November 2017, pp. 3205–12.

107 This section on Syria has been drawn from two key reports: Aula Abbara et al., 'Antimicrobial Resistance in the Context of the Syrian Conflict: Drivers Before and After the Onset of Conflict and Key Recommendations', in *International Journal of Infectious Diseases*, Vol. 73, August 2018, pp. 1–6; Aula Abbara et al., 'A summary and Appraisal of Existing Evidence of Antimicrobial Resistance in the

Syrian Conflict', in *International Journal of Infectious* Diseases, Vol. 75, October 2018, pp. 26–33.

108 D. Kutaini and C. Davila, 'Pharmaceutical Industry in Syria', in *Journal of Medicine and Life*, Vol. 3, No. 3, July–September 2010, pp. 348–50. See also 'Crisis in Syria hits pharma industry and drug supplies', *Pharmaceutical Technology*, 10 February 2013, https://www.pharmaceutical-technology.com/uncategorised/newscrisis-in-syria-hits-pharma-industry-and-drug-supplies/.

109 Omar Dewachi, Skelton et al., 'Changing Therapeutic Geographies of the Iraqi and Syrian Wars', in the *Lancet* series: *Health in the Arab World: A View from Within*, Vol. 383, No. 9915, 1 February 2014.

110 'Antibiotic Resistance – Tackling a Danger of a Different Kind in the Syrian Arab Republic', World Health Organization, 1 November 2017, https://www.who.int/news-room/feature-stories/detail/anti-biotic-resistance-tackling-a-danger-of-a-different-kind-in-the-syr-ian-arab-republic.

111 O.J. Dyar et al., on behalf of ESGAP (ESCMID Study Group for Antimicrobial Stewardship), 'What is antimicrobial stewardship?' in *Clinical Microbiology and Infection* Vol. 23, No. 11, p. 796.

112 E. Charani et al., 'An Analysis of the Development and Implementation of a Smartphone Application for the Delivery of Antimicrobial Prescribing Policy: Lessons Learnt', in *Journal of Antimicrobial Chemotherapy*, Vol. 68, No. 4, April 2013.

113 E. Charani et al., 'The Differences in Antibiotic Decision-making between Acute Surgical and Acute Medical Teams: An Ethnographic Study of Culture and Team Dynamics', in *Clinical Infectious Diseases*, Vol. 69, No. 1, 1 July 2019.

114 Dafna Yahav et al., 'Seven Versus 14 Days of Antibiotic Therapy for Uncomplicated Gram-negative Bacteremia: A Noninferiority Randomized Controlled Trial', in *Clinical Infectious Diseases*, Vol. 69, No. 7, 1 October, 2019.

115   Emma Wilkinson, 'No Going Back: how the Pandemic is Changing Hospital Pharmacy', in *Pharmaceutical Journal*, 2 July 2020.

116   Matthew Jones, 'On the Frontline of Antibiotic Resistance in South Sudan', Longitude Prize, 18 April 2018, https://longitudeprize.org/blog-post/frontline-antibiotic-resistance-south-sudan.

117   Marian Knight et al., 'Prophylactic Antibiotics in the Prevention of Infection After Operative Vaginal Delivery (ANODE): A Multi-centre Randomised Controlled Trial', in the *Lancet*, Vol. 393, No. 10189, 15 June 2019; Jeremy D. Keenan et al., for the MORDOR Study Group, 'Azithromycin to Reduce Childhood Mortality in Sub-Saharan Africa', in *New England Journal of Medicine* Vol. 378, No. 17, 26 April 2018, pp. 1583–92.

118   Kim Lewis, 'Programmed Death in Bacteria', in *Microbiology and Molecular Biology Reviews*, Vol. 64, No. 3, September 2000.

119   Michael E. Chirgwin et al., 'Novel Therapeutic Strategies Applied to *Pseudomonas aeruginosa* Infections in Cystic Fibrosis', in *Materials*, December 2019.

120   Jiangdong Huo et al., 'Neutralizing Nanobodies Bind SARS-CoV-2 Spike RBD and Block Interaction with ACE2', in *Nature: Structural and Molecular Biology*, 13 July 2020.

121   Rachell Babb and Liise-Anne Pirofski, 'Help is on the Way: Monoclonal Antibody Therapy for Multi-Drug Resistant Bacteria', in *Virulence*, Vol. 8, No. 7, October 2017.

122   Zachariah DeFilipp et al., 'Drug-Resistant *E. coli* Bacteremia Transmitted by Fecal Microbiota Transplant', in *New England Journal of Medicine*, 21 November 2019.

123   Although beautiful images of microbiome components are available from the work of Martin Oeggerli, a Swiss microbiologist. See *National Geographic*, January 2020.

124   Andrew Maltez Thomas and Nicola Segata, 'Multiple Levels of the Unknown in Microbiome Research', in *BMC Biology*, Vol. 17, No. 48, 12 June 2019.

125 For example: Renick, Jovanovic, Roche et al., 'The Topical Metallo-protease SN514 Enhances Antimicrobial Activity against Bacterial Biofilms', prepublication presentation at MHSRS, 2019; Baugh, Philips, Ekanayaka, Piddock, et al., 'Inhibition of Multidrug Efflux as a Strategy to Prevent Biofilm Formation', in *Journal of Antimicrobial Chemotherapy*, Vol. 69, No. 3, 31 October 2013, pp. 673–81; and many other almost entirely incomprehensible papers about under-mining biofilm resistance.

126 Great summary, great science communication: see Jonathan Otter et al., *Smart Surfaces to Tackle Infection and Antimicrobial Resistance*, Briefing Paper No. 4, Institute for Molecular Science and Engineering, Imperial College London, March 2020.

127 Jonathan M. Stokes et al., 'A Deep Learning Approach to Antibiotic Discovery', in *Cell*, Vol. 180, No. 4, pp. 688–702, February 2020.

128 See GARDP webinar, 'Putting children first in the fight against antibiotic resistance', 25 June 2020; and the GARDP 'In Focus' document, 'Making Children's Antibiotics a Priority', May 2020.

129 Joseph A. Lewnard et al., 'Childhood Vaccines and Antibiotic Use in Low- and Middle-income Countries', in *Nature*, Vol. 581, 29 April 2020.

130 'How WHO Is Supporting Ongoing Vaccination Efforts during The COVID-19 Pandemic', World Health Organization, 14 July 2020, https://www.who.int/news-room/feature-stories/detail/how-who-is-supporting-ongoing-vaccination-efforts-during-the-covid-19-pandemic.

131 Stats from the Gavi Vaccine Alliance, *Protect, Prevent, Prosper*; and 'Harvest for the World', The Isley Brothers.

132 Charles Clift, 'Review of Progress on Antimicrobial Resistance', Centre on Global Health Security, Chatham House, October 2019, p. 15.

133 See 'GARDP Receives Additional Funding from Germany to

Tackle Drug-Resistant Hospital Infections', in GARP press release, 17 September 2020, https://gardp.org/news-resources/gardp-receives-additional-funding-germany/.

134 Sameer S. Kadri and Helen W. Boucher, 'US Efforts to Curb Antibiotic Resistance – Are We Saving Lives?', in *New England Journal of Medicine*, 27 August 2020.

135 See Marc Mendelson et al., 'Antibiotic Resistance Has a Language Problem', in *Nature*, Vol. 545, p. 23, May 2017.

PART THREE: FAMINE

136 See Merlin Sheldrake, *Entangled Life* (London: Bodley Head, 2020), for instance.

137 Onions, for instance. Sang Hye Ji, Tae Kwang Kim et al., 'The Major Postharvest Disease of Onion and Its Control with Thymol Fumigation During Low-Temperature Storage', in *Mycobiology* Vol. 46, No. 3, September 2018, pp. 242–53.

138 Matthew C. Fisher et al., 'Worldwide Emergence of Resistance to Antifungal Drugs Challenges Human Health and Food Security', in *Science*, Vol. 360, No. 6390, 18 May 2018; Deepak K. Ray et al., 'Recent Patterns of Crop Yield Growth and Stagnation', in *Nature Communications*, Vol. 3, No. 1293, 18 December 2012.

139 David Moore, *Fungal Biology in the Origin and Emergence of Life* (Cambridge: Cambridge University Press, 2013), p. 5.

140 Tara Djokic et al., 'Earliest Signs of Life in Land Preserved in Ca. 3.5 Ga Hot Spring Deposits', in *Nature Communications*, Vol. 8, No. 15263, 9 May 2017.

141 David Moore, *Fungal Biology in the Origin and Emergence of Life*.

142 J. W. Deacon, *Fungal Biology* (London: Blackwell Publishing, 2006), pp. 12–35.

143 Ibid., p. 31.

144   E. C. Large, *Advance of the Fungi* (New York: H. Holt & Co., 1940), p. 39.

145   John Dighton, Tatyana Tugay and Nelli Zhdanova, 'Fungi and Ionizing Radiation from Radionuclides', in *FEMS Microbiology Letters* Vol. 281, No. 2, April 2008, pp. 109–20.

146   David Soll, 'The Ins and Outs of DNA Fingerprinting the Infectious Fungi', in *Clinical Microbiology Reviews* Vol. 13, No. 2, April 2000, pp. 332–70.

147   Kimberley Jane May and Jean Beagle Ristaino, 'Identity of the mt DNA Haplotype(s) of Phytophthora infestans in Historical Specimens from the Irish Potato Famine', in *Mycological Research* Vol. 108, No. 5, May 2004, pp. 471–9.

148   Meredith D. M. Jones et al., 'Discovery of Novel Intermediate Forms Redefines the Fungal Tree of Life', in *Nature* Vol. 474, May 2011, pp. 200–3.

149   May and Ristaino, 'Identity of the mtDNA haplotype(s) of Phytophthora infestans in Historical Specimens from the Irish Potato Famine'.

150   http://botanicgardens.ie/science-and-learning/the-national-herbarium/

151   Ayush Pathak et al., 'Comparative Genomics of Alexander Fleming's Original *Penicillium* Isolate (IMI 15378) Reveals Sequence Divergence of Penicillin Synthesis Genes', in *Scientific Reports* Vol. 10, No. 15705, 24 September 2020.

152   See Murra, Mayer and Fonseca, cited in the bibliography of John Earls, 'The Character of Inca and Andean Agriculture', Departamento de Ciencias Sociales, Pontificia Universidad Católica del Perú. Also, Ramiro Matos Mendieta, *The Great Inka Road: Engineering an Empire* (Washington, DC: Smithsonian Books, 2015); and Marcel Mazoyer and Laurence Roudart, *A History of World Agriculture* (EarthScan-Routledge, 2006), pp. 206–10.

153   https://cipotato.org/about/.

154 Erik Stokstad, 'This Spud's For You: A Breeding Revolution Could Unleash the Potential of Potato', in *Science*, 7 February 2019.

155 W. Rapin et al., 'An Interval of High Salinity in Ancient Gale Crater Lake on Mars', in *Nature Geoscience* Vol. 12, 7 October 2019.

156 See the video at https://cipotato.org/annualreport2016/stories/mars-potatoes/.

157 Jan W. Low et al., 'Nutrient-Dense Orange-Fleshed Sweetpotato: Advances in Drought-Tolerance Breeding and Understanding of Management Practices for Sustainable Next-Generation Cropping Systems in Sub-Saharan Africa', in *Frontiers in Sustainable Food Systems*, 12 May 2020, https://doi.org/10.3389/fsufs.2020.00050.

158 'Revised Strategy and Corporate Plan 2014–2023', CIP, https://cipotato.org/about/corporate-plan/.

159 Hugo Campos and Oscar Ortiz (eds), *The Potato Crop* (Cham: Springer, 2020).

160 Christian W. B. Bachem, Herman J. van Eck and Michiel E. de Vries, 'Understanding Genetic Load in Potato for Hybrid Diploid Breeding', in *Molecular Plant: Spotlight* Vol. 12, No. 7, 1 July 2019.

161 Erik Stokstad, 'The Famine Fighter's Last Battle', in *Science*, Vol. 324, No. 5928, 8 May 2009.

162 'Norman Borlaug: Biographical', Nobel Peace Prize 1970, https://www.nobelprize.org/prizes/peace/1970/borlaug/biographical/.

163 See MARDy, the Mycology Antifungal Resistance Database, Twitter: @MARDYfungi; and MinION and SmidgION by Oxford Nanopore Technologies.

164 Günter Theissen, 'The Proper Place of Hopeful Monsters in Evolutionary Biology', in *Theory in Biosciences* Vol. 124, March 2006, pp. 349–69.

165 Mikhail Katsnelson, Yuri Wolf and Eugene Koonin, 'On the Feasibility of Salvational Evolution', posted to bioRxiv preprint server for comments, 23 August 2018.

166 M. S. Hovmøller et al., 'Replacement of the European Wheat Yellow

Rust Population by New Races from the Centre of Diversity in the Near-Himalayan Region', in *Plant Pathology* Vol. 65, No. 3, April 2016, pp. 402–11.

167 For a really good explanation of GM crops and technology, see 'GM Plants: Questions and Answers', published by the Royal Society, May 2016.

168 Randy Ploetz, 'Panama Disease: A Classic and Destructive Disease of Banana', in *Plant Health Progress* Vol. 1, No. 1, 27 July 2018.

169 Mpoki W. Shimwela et al., 'Banana Xanthomonas Wilt Continues to Spread in Tanzania Despite an Intensive Symptomatic Plant Removal Campaign: An Impending Socio-Economic and Ecological Disaster', in *Food Security* Vol. 8, 16 September 2016, pp. 939–51.

170 www.amphibianark.org.

171 See Matthew C. Fisher and Trenton W. J. Garner, 'Chytrid Fungi and Global Amphibian Declines', in *Nature Reviews Microbiology* Vol. 18, No. 6, 25 February 2020.

172 David S. Blehert et al., 'Bat White-Nose Syndrome: An Emerging Fungal Pathogen?' in *Science* Vol. 323, No. 5911, 9 January 2009.

173 Professor Matt Fisher, quoted in Becky Allen, 'Antifungal Resistance', in *Imperial* 47, Winter 2019/20.

174 L. Huang, et al., 'Invasive Pulmonary Aspergillosis in Patients with Influenza Infection: A Retrospective Study and Review of the Literature', in *Clinical Respiratory Journal* Vol. 13, No. 4, April 2019, pp. 202–11.

175 Jacques F. Meis et al., 'Clinical Implications of Globally Emerging Azole Resistance in *Aspergillus Fumigatus*', in *Philosophical Transactions B* Vol. 371, No. 1709, 5 December 2016.

176 Thomas R. Sewell et al., 'Elevated Prevalence of Azole-Resistant *Aspergillus fumigatus* in Urban versus Rural Environments in the United Kingdom', in *Antimicrobial Agents and Chemotherapy* Vol. 63, No. 9, September 2019.

177 Disclosure: one company, Pulmocide, working on this delivery mech-

anism is based at Imperial College London. I have no financial interest in this company, but if they get it right, we will all look good.

178 Meis et al., 'Clinical Implications of Globally Emerging Azole Resistance in *Aspergillus Fumigatus*'.

179 L. Weaver, H. T. Michels and C. W. Keevil, 'Potential for Preventing Spread of Fungi in Air-Conditioning Systems Constructed Using Copper Instead of Aluminium', in *Letters in Applied Microbiology* Vol. 50, No. 1, January 2010.

180 Gagandeep Gohlar and Stephen Hughes, 'How to Improve Anti-fungal Stewardship', in *Pharmaceutical Journal,* 19 July 2019.

181 R. W. Schneider et al., 'First Report of Soybean Rust Caused by Phakopsora pachyrhizi in the Continental United States', in *Plant Disease* Vol. 89, No. 7, July 2005.

182 See Tamara Lucas and Richard Horton, 'The 21st-Century Great Food Transformation', in the *Lancet* Vol. 393, No. 10170, 2 February 2019; L. Wen, C. R. Bowen and G. L. Hartman, 'Prediction of Short-Distance Aerial Movement of Phakopsora Pachyrhizi Urediniospores Using Machine Learning', in *Phytopathology* Vol. 107, No. 10, October 2017, pp. 1187–98. See also D. A. Shah et al., 'Predicting Plant Disease Epidemics from Functionally Represented Weather Series', in *Philosophical Transactions B* Vol. 374, No. 1775, 24 June 2019.

183 M. Meyer et al., 'Quantifying Airborne Dispersal Routes of Pathogens over Continents to Safeguard Global Wheat Supply', in *Nature Plants* Vol. 3, October 2017, p. 781.

184 Adel Aldaghbashy, 'Wheat Plague Spreading through Yemen', in *SciDev.Net*, 1 February 2018.

185 'Gene Discovery May Halt Worldwide Wheat Epidemic', in *Science Daily*, 16 November 2017.

186 A. P. Sturman, P. D. Tyson and P. C. D'Abreton, 'A Preliminary Study of the Transport of Air from Africa and Australia to New Zealand', in *Journal of the Royal Society of New Zealand* Vol. 27, No.

4, pp. 485–98; Matthew C. Fisher et al., 'Emerging Fungal Threats to Animal, Plant and Ecosystem Health', in *Nature* Vol. 484, No. 7393, 11 April 2012, p. 191.

187 Paolo Gonthier et al., 'Pathogen Introduction as a Collateral Effect of Military Activity', in *Mycological Research* Vol.108, No. 5, May 2004, p. 470.

188 See J. R. Hale, *War and Society in Renaissance Europe* (Baltimore, MD: Johns Hopkins University Press, 1986), pp. 191–6.

189 UN Meetings Coverage press release: 'Adopting Resolution 2417 (2018), Security Council Strongly Condemns Starving of Civilians, Unlawfully Denying Humanitarian Access as Warfare Tactics', 24 May 2018.

190 PAX, Siege Watch: https://siegewatch.org.

191 Grace J. Carroll et al., 'Evaluation of Nutrition Interventions in Children in Conflict Zones: A Narrative Review', in *Advances in Nutrition* Vol. 8, No. 5, September 2017, p. 773.

192 André Briend, 'The Complex Relationship Between Wasting and Stunting', in *American Journal of Clinical Nutrition* Vol. 110, No. 2, August 2019.

193 Andrew J. Prendergast and Jean H. Humphrey, 'The Stunting Syndrome in Developing Countries', in *Paediatrics and International Child Health* Vol. 34, No. 4, October 2014. For the call to improve metrics, see Jonathan C. K. Wells et al., 'Beyond Wasted and Stunted – A Major Shift to Fight Child Nutrition', in the *Lancet: Child and Adolescent Health* Vol. 3, No. 11, 1 November 2019.

194 Simon M. Schoenbuchner et al., 'The Relationship between Wasting and Stunting: A Retrospective Cohort Analysis of Longitudinal Data in Gambian Children from 1976 to 2016', in *American Journal of Clinical Nutrition* Vol. 110, No. 2, August 2019, pp. 498–507.

195 Lewis Wolpert, *How We Live and Why We Die* (London: Faber & Faber, 2010), p. 140.

196 Natasha Lelijveld et al., 'Long-term Effects of Severe Acute Malnu-

trition on Lung Function in Malawian Children: A Cohort Study',
in *European Respiratory Journal* Vol. 49, No. 4, 2017.

197 Claire D. Bourke, James A. Berkley and Andrew J. Prendergast,
'Immune Dysfunction as a Cause and Consequence of Malnutrition', in *Trends in Immunology* Vol. 37, No. 6, June 2016.

198 Rosemarie De Weirdt and Tom Van de Wiele, 'Micromanagement
in the Gut: Microenvironmental Factors Govern Colon Mucosal
Biofilm Structure and Functionality', in *NPJ Biofilms and Microbiomes* Vol. 1, October 2015.

199 Bourke, Berkley and Prendergast, 'Immune Dysfunction as a Cause
and Consequence of Malnutrition'.

200 Andrew J. Prendergast et al., 'Stunting is Characterized by Chronic
Inflammation in Zimbabwean Infants', in *PLoS One* Vol. 9, No. 2,
February 2014.

201 Bourke, Berkley and Prendergast, 'Immune Dysfunction as a Cause
and Consequence of Malnutrition', p. 386.

202 'Executive Summary', *Global Nutrition Report 2018*, p. 19.

203 André Devaux et al., 'Global Food Security, Contributions from
Sustainable Potato Agri-Food Systems', in Campos and Ortiz (eds.),
The Potato Crop.

204 Emma Pomeroy et al., 'Trade-Offs in Relative Limb Length among
Peruvian Children: Extending the Thrifty Phenotype Hypothesis to
Limb Proportions', in *PLoS One* Vol. 7, No. 12, December 2012.

205 *The Paediatric Blast Injury Field Manual* (Imperial College London,
2019 (open access)), p. 25, Appendix on p. 43.

206 John Milwood Hargrave et al., 'Blast Injuries in children: A Mixed-
Methods Narrative Review', in *BMJ Paediatrics Open* Vol. 3, No. 1,
2019.

207 Bettina Sederquist et al., 'Recent Research on the Growth Plate:
Impact of Inflammatory Cytokines on Longitudinal Bone Growth',
in *Journal of Molecular Endocrinology* Vol. 53, No. 1, October 2014.

208 'Growth Plate Injuries', National Institute of Arthritis and Musculo-

skeletal and Skin Diseases, https://www.niams.nih.gov/health-topics/growth-plate-injuries.

209   Amy K. Hegarty et al., 'Evaluation of a Method to Scale Muscle Strength for Gait Simulations of Children with Cerebral Palsy', in *Journal of Biomechanics* Vol. 83, 23 January 2019.

210   Prendergast and Humphrey, 'The Stunting Syndrome in Developing Countries', p. 257 and bibliographical references.

211   Lisa Jones et al., 'Prevalence and Risk of Violence against Children with Disabilities: A Systematic Review and Meta-Analysis of Observational Studies', in the *Lancet* Vol. 380, No. 9845, 8 September 2012.

212   Helen Young et al., 'Public Nutrition in Complex Emergencies', in the *Lancet,* Vol. 364, No. 9448, 20 November 2004.

213   Alex C. Dela Cuadra, 'The Philippine Micronutrient Supplementation Programme', in *Food and Nutrition Bulletin* Vol. 21, No. 4, January 2000, p. 512.

214   Carroll et al., 'Evaluation of Nutrition Interventions in Children in Conflict Zones: A Narrative Review'.

215   'The Double Burden of Malnutrition', series from the *Lancet* journals, 16 December 2019.

216   See 'Child and Adolescent: Health and Development', part of the World Bank series, November 2017. See H. Luz McNaughton Reyes et al., 'Adolescent Dating Violence Prevention Programmes: A Global Systematic Review of Evaluation Studies', in *Lancet: Child and Adolescent Health*, 19 November 2020, https://www.thelancet.com/journals/lanchi/article/PIIS2352-4642(20)30276-5/fulltext. See also Lindsay Stark, Ilana Seff and Chen Reis, 'Gender-Based Violence Against Adolescent Girls in Humanitarian Settings: A Review of the Evidence', in *Lancet: Child and Adolescent Health*, 19 November 2020, https://www.thelancet.com/journals/lanchi/article/PIIS2352-4642(20)30245-5/fulltext.

217   P. Christian and E. R. Smith, 'Adolescent Undernutrition: Global

Burden, Physiology, and Nutritional Risks', in *Annals of Nutrition and Metabolism* Vol. 72, No. 4, May 2018, pp. 316–28. See also Youn Hee Jee et al., 'Malnutrition and Catch-Up Growth During Childhood and Puberty', in *World Review of Nutrition and Dietetics* Vol. 109, January 2014, pp. 89–100.

218 Andrew M. Prentice et al., 'Critical Windows for Nutritional Interventions against Stunting', in *American Journal of Clinical Nutrition* Vol. 97, No. 5, May 2013, pp. 911–18.

219 Elizabeth L. et al., 'Do Effects of Early Life Interventions on Linear Growth Correspond to Effects on Neurobehavioural Development? A Systematic Review and Meta-Analysis', in the *Lancet: Global Health* Vol. 7, No. 10, October 2019.

220 Mike L. T. Berendsen et al., 'Non-specific Effects of Vaccines and Stunting: Timing May Be Essential', in *EBioMedicine* Vol. 8, 1 June 2016, pp. 341–8. Mahrrouz Caputo et al., 'Vaccinations and Infections Are Associated With Unrelated Antibody Titers', in *Frontiers in Pediatrics* Vol. 7, No. 254, 25 June 2019.

221 Trevor Duke, 'What the PERCH Study Means for Future Pneumonia Strategies', in the *Lancet* Vol. 394, No. 10200, 31 August 2019.

222 Velislava N. Petrova et al., 'Incomplete Genetic Reconstruction of B Cell Pools Contributes to Prolonged Immunosuppression after Measles', in *Science Immunology* Vol. 4, No. 41, 29 November 2019.

223 Andrew Prendergast, 'Malnutrition and Vaccination in Developing Countries', in *Philosophical Transactions B* Vol. 370, No. 1671, 19 June 2015.

224 'Mosul Recovery: Honey Production in Mosul Reaches a Record 48,000 kilograms', Mosul Eye, 11 January 2019.

225 Beekeepers had other things to do during the occupation. See Dunya Mikhail, *The Beekeeper of Sinjar: Rescuing the Stolen Women of Iraq* (London: Serpents Tail, 2019).

PART FOUR: DEATH

226   Although the very first person to ask me was Rebecca Fogg.

227   Ian Twiddy, 'Visions of Reconciliation: Longley, Heaney and the Greeks', in *Irish Studies Review* Vol. 21, No. 4, November 2013, pp. 425–43.

228   Michael Longley, 'Ceasefire', in *Collected Poems* (London: Jonathan Cape, 2007).

229   Sophocles, *Antigone*, 2012 National Theatre production (UK), with Jodie Whittaker as Antigone, translation by Don Taylor, 1986.

230   Hiroo Kanamori, 'Lessons from the 2004 Sumatra–Andaman Earthquake', in *Philosophical Transactions A* Vol. 364, 15 August 2006, p. 1940.

231   Yuichiro Tanioka et al., 'Rupture Process of the 2004 Great Sumatra–Andaman Earthquake Estimated from Tsunami Waveforms', in *Earth, Planets and Space* Vol. 58, No. 2, February 2006, pp. 203–9; Thorne Lay et al., 'The Great Sumatra–Andaman Earthquake of 26 December 2004', in *Science* Vol. 308, No. 5725, 20 May 2005, pp. 1127–33.

232   See Jonathan M. Katz, *The Big Truck That Went By* (London: Palgrave Macmillan, 2013).

233   From the 'Overview' of the Study of the Tsunami Aftermath and Recovery (STAR), http://stardata.org.

234   Elizabeth Frankenberg et al. 'Mortality, the Family and the Indian Ocean Tsunami', in *Economic Journal* Vol. 121, No. 554, August 2011, pp. 162–8.

235   Thomas W. Gillespie et al. 'Night-Time Lights Time Series of Tsunami Damage, Recovery, and Economic Metrics in Sumatra, Indonesia', in *Remote Sensing Letters* Vol. 5, No. 3, January 2014, pp. 286–94.

236   Emile Okal et al., 'Oman Field Survey after the December 2004 Indian Ocean Tsunami', in *Earthquake Spectra* Vol. 22, No. 3,

June 2006. Also author interviews with Stefan Eiker and Gavin Houghton.

237 Hermann M. Fritz and Emile Okal, 'Yemen: Socotra Field Survey of the 2004 Indian Ocean Tsunami', UNESCO-IOC post-tsunami survey, December 2006.

238 Oliver W. Morgan et al., 'Mass Fatality Management following South Asian Tsunami Disaster: Case Studies in Thailand, Indonesia, and Sri Lanka', in *PLoS Med*, Vol. 3, No. 6, June 2006, pp. 809–15.

239 John Cosgrave, 'Synthesis Report: Expanded Summary. Joint Evaluation of the International Response to the Indian Ocean Tsunami', Tsunami Evaluation Coalition, January 2007, p. 5.

240 'Ten Key Lessons for OCHA: The Tsunami Evaluation Coalition, the South Asia Earthquake and the Lebanon Crisis', in *OCHA Annual Report, 2006*, United Nations, p. 32.

241 Interpol Tsunami Evaluation Working Group, 'The DVI Response to the South East Asian Tsunami between December 2004 and February 2006', compiled by Derek Forest, Interpol/Thai Tsunami Victim Identification.

242 This section is drawn from Cordner and Tidball-Binz, 'Humanitarian Forensic Action – Its Origins and Future', in *Forensic Science International* Vol. 279, October 2017, pp. 65–71. Also, 'Using Forensic Science to Care for the Dead and Search for the Missing: In conversation with Dr Morris Tidball-Binz', in *International Review of the Red Cross* Vol. 99, No. 905, August 2017, pp. 689–707.

243 The most up-to-date statement on this by the ICRC was issued in August 2019: *Humanity after Life: Respecting and Protecting the Dead.*

244 Ibid.

245 Ahmed Al-Dawoody, 'Management of the Dead from the Islamic law and International Humanitarian Law Perspectives', in *International Review of the Red Cross* Vol. 99, No. 2, 'The Missing' themed issue, August 2017, pp. 759–84.

246 'Using Forensic Science to Care for the Dead and Search for the

Missing: In Conversation with Morris Tidball-Binz', in Roberto C. Parra, Sara C. Zapico and Douglas H. Ubelaker (eds.), *Forensic Science and Humanitarian Action: Interacting with the Dead and the Living* (London: John Wiley, 2020).

247 Stephen Cordner and Sarah Ellingham, 'Two Halves Make a Whole: Both First Responders and Experts Are Needed for the Management and Identification of the Dead in Large Disasters', in *Forensic Science International* Vol. 279, October 2017, pp. 60–4.

248 Cordner, Coninx, Kim, van Alphen and Tidball-Binz (eds.), *Management of Dead Bodies after Disasters: A Field Manual for First Responders* (Geneva: ICRC, WHO, PAHO, IFRC, Second Edition, 2016).

249 Martin Schneider, François Chappuis and Sophie Pautex, 'How Do Expatriate Health Workers Cope with Needs to Provide Palliative Care in Humanitarian Emergency Assistance? A Qualitative Study with in-depth interviews', in *Palliative Medicine* Vol. 32, No. 10, 16 August 2018, pp. 1567–74.

250 Stephen Cordner, Heinrich Bouwer and Morris Tidball-Binz, 'The Ebola Epidemic in Liberia and Managing the Dead – A Future Role for Humanitarian Forensic Action?' in *Forensic Science International* Vol. 279, October 2017, p. 304.

251 Ibid, pp. 302–9.

252 Oran Finegan et al., 'ICRC: General Guidance for the Management of the Dead Related to COVID-19', in *Forensic Science International: Synergy* Vol. 2, 31 March 2020, p. 134.

253 Subarna Roy et al. 'Acute Diarrhea in Children after 2004 Tsunami, Andaman Islands', in *Emerging Infectious Diseases* Vol. 15, No. 5, May 2009, pp. 849.

254 *Ten Years After the Tsunami of 2004: Impact, Action, Change, Future* (WHO Publications, 2015).

255 Jean-Christophe Gaillard et al., 'Ethnic Groups' Response to the 26 December 2004 Earthquake and Tsunami in Aceh, Indonesia', in *Natural Hazards* Vol. 47, No. 1, October 2008, pp. 17–38.

256 Esther Pan, 'Indonesia: The Aceh Peace Agreement', Council on Foreign Relations, 15 September 2005, www.cfr.org/backgrounder/indonesia-aceh-peace-agreement.

257 Frankenberg et al., 'Mortality, the Family and the Indian Ocean Tsunami'.

258 Duncan Thomas et al. 'Effect of Stress on Cardiometabolic Health 12 Years after the Indian Ocean Tsunami: A Quasi-Experimental Longitudinal Study', in the *Lancet: Planetary Health* Vol. 2, No. 1, 28 May 2018, p. 8.

259 Elizabeth Frankenberg et al., *Study of the Tsunami Aftermath and Recovery (STAR): Study Design and Results*, STAR, 17 April 2020, http://stardata.org/st_files/STARdesignresults.pdf.

260 MDF-JRF Secretariat, *The Multi Donor Fund for Aceh and Nias: A Framework for Reconstruction through Effective Partnerships*, MDF-JRF working paper series no. 5, World Bank, Jakarta, 2012, p. 50. See Jennifer Hyndman, *Dual Disasters: Humanitarian Aid After the Tsunami* (Sterling, VA: Kumarian Press, 2011) for an explanation of the ethnic divisions in Aceh and beyond.

261 Edward Aspinall, 'Peace Without Justice? The Helsinki Peace Process in Aceh', Centre for Humanitarian Dialogue, Switzerland, April 2008. See also, 'Aceh Peace Process Follow-Up Project: Final Report', Crisis Management Initiative, 2012.

262 https://www.bbc.co.uk/news/world-asia-55846699: 'LGBT rights: Indonesia's Aceh flogs two men for having sex.'

263 Tim Folger, 'Will Indonesia Be Ready for the Next Tsunami?', in *National Geographic*, 28 September 2018 (originally published 26 December 2014), https://www.nationalgeographic.com/news/2018/9/141226-tsunami-indonesia-catastrophe-banda-aceh-warning-science/.

264 Oran Finegan et al., 'ICRC: General Guidance for the Management of the Dead Related to COVID-19', in *Forensic Science International: Synergy* Vol. 2, 31 March 2020, pp. 129–37.

Acknowledgements

Aula Abarra

Leah Adamson

Maisam Al-ahmed

Christina Aahlefeldt Laurvig

Jaime Aguilera Garcia

Tahlil Ahmed

Michael Almond

Bashar Alsuofi

Jon Alvis

Rich Arcus

Roderick Bailey

Simon Baker

Manica Balasegaram

Hanan Balkhy

Michael Bertaume

Tamiko Bolton Soros

Arij Bourlesan-Skelton

Claire Bourke

Steve Bree

Martin Bricknell

Bram Broerse

Kieran Brophy

Amanda Brydon

Anthony Bull

Gilbert Burnham

Jeremy Cannon

Tom Catena

Esmita Charani

Michael Coates

Andrew Czyzewski

Tom Davies

James Denselow

Christian Dinesen

Sarah Dixon Smith

Sabine van Elsland

Eva van Esschoten

Nisha Fazal

Rebecca Fogg

Lucy Foss

Iain Gibb

Claire Green

Derek Gregory

Kirby Gross

Sarah Gurr

Phoebe Harkins

David Henson

Shehan Hettiaratchy

Tuuli Hongisto

Chih-Hsing Huang

Barbara Holcomb

Simon Horne

Mohammed Jawad

Ellie Johnston

Craig Jones

Rob Iliffe

Anna Kampmann

Natasha Kaplinsky

Mark Kaye

Jakob Kopperud

Peter Le Feuvre

Guy Martin

Spyros Masouros

Elizabeth Masters

Elizabeth Macaulay

Ross Macfarlane

Aicha Merez

John Milwood Hargrave

Omar Mohammed

Martin Moody

John McCarthy

Michael McCourt

Robbie McIntyre

Ana McLaughlin

Charles Montagu

David Nabarro

Chris Natt

Christine Norman

Catrin Nye

Christina Obiero

Andi Orlowski

Jon Otter

Caro Parker

Jasmine Palmer

Harry Parker

Imogen Pelham

Joe Penfield

Stefan Peterson

Joe Piper

Maryam Philpott

Laura Piddock

The Potato Projecteers

Alex Potter

Andrew Prendergast

Todd Rasmussen

Jon Riley

Rowan Riley

Victor Riitho

Ruairi Robertson

Paul Reavley

Keyan Salarkia

Bob Seddon

Sally Sheard

Anne Silverman

Peter Skelton

Paul Spiegel

Michael Stanes

Matt Sztajnkrycer

Dan Stinner

Christopher Stoltz

Rowan Story

Emma Sykes

Nigel Tai

Morris Tidball-Binz

Scott Veale

Michael von Bertele

Amanda Wallace

Kevin Watkins

James Watt

Paul Wise

Sara Wolper

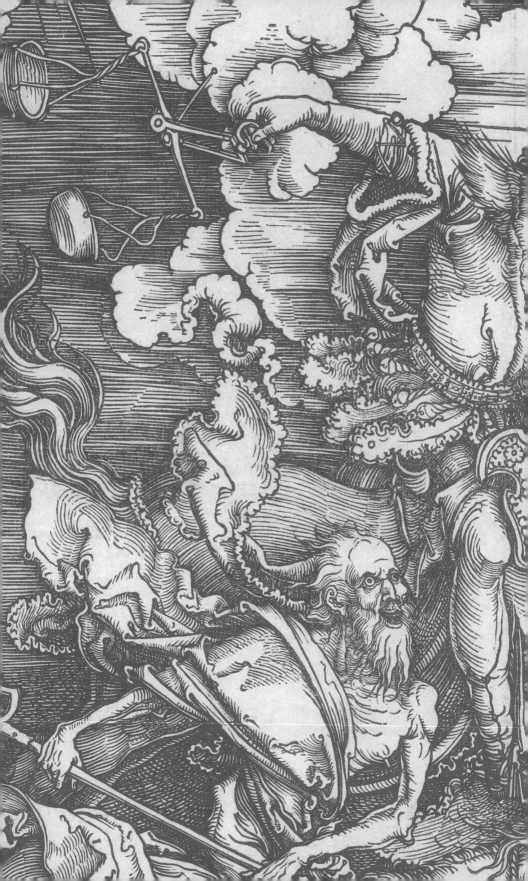